Let's Have A Quickie!
Simple Sex Education

Matthew Williams, LCSW

ISBN: 979-8-9995246-1-4

To my wife who shares my interest in all things sexy.

CONTENTS

About The Author

About the Author

The author has a Master's degree in Social Work, specializing in mental health. He has been practicing psychotherapy since 2008 and teaching Social Work at Sacramento State University since 2015. The inspiration for this book was originally a brief lecture he put together for his students during their LGBTQ segment. He wanted to add a little more depth to the original curriculum. What quickly became apparent, however, was that there was far more valuable information than would fit in that segment alone.

This booklet represents a comprehensive collection of insights on sex and sexuality, packaged for accessibility and practical application. The content draws from years of professional experience, academic research, and ongoing learning. The author is passionate about demystifying these topics and believes that better understanding leads to better experiences.

For readers wanting to explore specific areas more deeply, you'll find a curated list of resources at the back of this booklet. These include podcasts, books, websites, and articles that can help you dive further into whatever aspects of sexuality spark your curiosity or interest. Whether you're looking to expand your knowledge, improve your relationships, or simply understand yourself better, these additional resources offer pathways for continued exploration.

Foreword

The Politics of Pleasure

As tempting as it is to say this book isn't political, that's simply not possible. The very act of discussing sexuality in America is inherently political. When I say that all people deserve sexual agency, pleasure, and respect, I'm making a statement that runs counter to powerful social and institutional forces.

Sex is political because access to sexual autonomy isn't distributed equally. Throughout history and continuing today, sexuality has been weaponized, restricted, and used as a means of control. Consider:

Sexual Violence: Rape, assault, harassment, and other non-consensual acts remain pervasive across societies. These aren't just individual crimes, but expressions of power imbalances embedded in our social structures.

Discrimination: People face vastly different treatment based on their sex, gender, and sexual orientation. From workplace harassment to healthcare barriers to legal restrictions, these inequalities shape who gets to experience sexuality freely and safely.

Reproductive Rights: Access to sex education, contraception, abortion, and maternal care remains deeply unequal and constantly under threat. The ability to control if, when, and how one becomes a parent is fundamental to sexual freedom.

Harmful Practices: Child marriage, genital mutilation, forced sterilization, purity culture, and conversion therapy continue globally. Each violates bodily autonomy in service of controlling sexuality.

Systemic Barriers: From discriminatory laws, religion, and biased cultural narratives about who "deserves" pleasure, these systems aren't accidents – they're designed to maintain certain power dynamics.

I'm not sharing this to depress you or to suggest that good sex requires a certain political affiliation. I'm acknowledging that when we talk about improving sexual experiences, we're swimming upstream against powerful currents that have shaped all of our attitudes about sex.

This doesn't mean we should view everyone with different sexual values as an enemy. In fact, that's counterproductive. My family motto is "don't be a dick," which might sound simplistic, but it contains genuine wisdom. It means approaching differences with curiosity rather than condemnation, recognizing that most people's attitudes, sexual and otherwise, were shaped by forces beyond their control.

The reality is that most of us are unlearning harmful messages about sex while trying to build healthier ones. That's not easy work, and it requires compassion, for ourselves and others. The political awareness I'm advocating isn't about picking fights but about understanding the larger context in which our most intimate experiences take place.

So yes, this book is political. But its politics are fundamentally about expanding freedom, pleasure, and connection for everyone; and I hope that's something we can all get behind, regardless of how we vote.

CHAPTER ONE

Consent

Consent: The Non-Negotiable Foundation

Don't let the brevity of this section belie its importance. There really isn't a whole lot you need to understand about consent, but what you do need to know is absolutely crucial. Here's the basics:

1. **It should be enthusiastic!** No one worth having sex with is okay having sex with someone who isn't really into it. It's not fun if you're not having fun, and it's not fun if your partner(s) aren't having fun. So if your potential partner has any hesitation, or if you yourself have a "wait, maybe" or an "I need more information" feeling, then it's a no. Silence is a no. A reluctant "okay" is a no. We're looking for a "fuck yeah!" vibe. Anything less is just not worth it.

2. **Unconscious is always a no.** Someone who is asleep or passed out cannot consent, period. (Some couples may role-play scenarios involving sleep or unconsciousness, but this requires explicit prior agreement when both parties are fully conscious and sober, clear boundaries, and established safe signals.)

3. **Severely drunk or high is a no.** Intoxication impairs judgment and the ability to give meaningful consent. A good rule: if someone is too drunk to drive, they're too drunk to consent to new sexual activities. Even if you've discussed scenarios involving alcohol beforehand, remember that extreme intoxication can prevent someone from using safe words or expressing discomfort.

4. **Consent applies to ALL interactions, not just sex acts.** Consent applies to touch, both sexual and non-sexual. It applies to every kind of interaction, including non-physical ones. If someone doesn't consent to having a conversation with you, then too bad buddy, the conversation is over. Respect extends to all forms of engagement.

5. **Consent is revocable at ANY time.** Even if you say "yes" in the beginning, you can still change your mind later. You don't like the shift in attitude, you suddenly aren't feeling the vibes, you just lost interest? Totally fine! Consent revoked and we bounce! No explanations required.

6. **Consent should be checked and rechecked.** Yes to one thing does NOT mean yes to all things. If you consented to oral and someone wants to do more, they should ask. If you're engaged in consensual activity and enthusiasm wanes, check in: "Are you still into this?" or "Do you want to try something else?" This is part of what makes communication during sex hot too!

7. **When in doubt, pause and check in.** If you're uncertain about your partner's consent, maybe their body language seems off or they've gone quiet, simply stop and ask. Better to briefly interrupt the moment than to risk violating someone's boundaries. The most confident lovers aren't afraid to confirm consent.

Remember: good consent practices aren't just about avoiding harm; they actually create the conditions for better, more connected sexual experiences. When everyone involved feels safe, respected, and genuinely wanted, that's when the really good stuff happens.

The Invisible Ingredient: Communication Is Your Best Sexual Skill

One of the hottest things you can do sexually is pay attention to your partner(s). Seriously. If you notice shifts in their enjoyment, pleasure, interest, or engagement and then check in and adjust accordingly - that's fucking hot! This attentiveness tells your partner(s) that you're genuinely interested in them and their enjoyment. It demonstrates that your pleasure is connected to them feeling seen, responded to, and desired - all elements that create profound sexual connection. Ideally, sex should be an equal opportunity feel-good experience for everyone involved.

But here in America, we make this surprisingly difficult. We send wildly contradictory messages about sex and sexuality. Sex remains a taboo topic, something "polite society" doesn't discuss openly, while simultaneously forming the foundation of countless advertising strategies. From products promising enhanced sexual performance to entire industries built around improving appearance to attract partners, we're swimming in sexual messaging while lacking the vocabulary to talk about it honestly.

The deeper cultural and historical reasons for this contradiction could fill another book entirely, but for our purposes, let's focus on the practical: communication is essential to good sex, full stop.

Consent is communicated. Safety is communicated. Personal desires, boundaries, and preferences for how one likes to be touched or engaged. All of this requires clear communication. Without it, we're essentially fumbling in the dark, hoping to accidentally stumble upon what works.

Most human communication is nonverbal. We can say all the "right" words, but tone, facial expressions, and body language often make a much stronger impact. That subtle tensing when you touch somewhere new, the slight change in breathing when something feels particularly good, the way eyes widen or close in response to sensation. These cues tell you far more than words alone.

That said, explicit verbal communication is still necessary, especially for consent to be crystal clear. "Does this feel good?" "Can I try something new?" "I'd love it if you would..." These phrases create space for both connection and boundary-setting. The same goes for "I don't like that," "a little to the left," "slow down," etc. The most attentive lovers balance their awareness of nonverbal cues with direct questions and clear statements.

In the chapters that follow, I'll discuss specific information for understanding the variety of sexual interactions we humans have. But the foundation of it all, the skill that elevates sex from mechanical to meaningful, is simply paying attention. It costs nothing, requires no special equipment, and yet transforms the entire experience for everyone involved.

CHAPTER TWO

What Are We Calling "Sex"?

What Do We Mean By "Sex"?

Sex is a multifaceted concept that encompasses biological, psychological, social, and cultural dimensions. At its most basic level, sex can refer to the biological classification of organisms—typically assigned at birth based on physical characteristics like chromosomes, hormones, and reproductive anatomy. However, even this classification is more complex than the traditional binary of male and female, as intersex variations demonstrate.

Sex also refers to physical intimacy and sexual activity, which varies widely across cultures, personal preferences, and relationship dynamics. It's a deeply personal experience that can involve pleasure, connection, exploration, and sometimes reproduction. In many societies, sex is shaped by norms, taboos, and power structures that influence how people experience and discuss it.

Beyond the physical, sex is intertwined with identity, relationships, and broader social narratives. How individuals define and experience sex is deeply influenced by their backgrounds, desires, and the contexts in which they live. A more inclusive understanding acknowledges that sex isn't just a biological function or a physical act; it's a complex interplay of personal, social, and political realities. While it's important to recognize this complexity, this booklet focuses primarily on the practical aspects of sexual activity; the different ways people connect physically and find pleasure with partners. By exploring various forms of sexual expression, we can better understand both the diversity of human sexuality and the common threads that connect our experiences. So let's dive into the how, what, and why of sexual activity with an open mind and a focus on mutual enjoyment.

The Mechanics of Sex: A Practical Guide to Sexual Activities

Whether you're new to sexual experiences, looking to expand your horizons, or just curious about what others might be doing, this guide breaks down common sexual activities. This is not meant to be a how-to manual, though there are some pro tips. See the resources section at the back for more in-depth information.

Remember: there's no "normal" or "required" way to have sex, and none of these acts are mandatory checkboxes on some universal sex list. What matters is consent, communication, and what brings pleasure to you and your partner(s).

Manual Stimulation: Getting Handsy

Hand-to-Vulva Play

Using hands to stimulate a vulva is often called fingering, rubbing, or manual stimulation. This can involve gently stroking the outer labia (the outer lips), circling or directly stimulating the clitoris (that sensitive bundle of nerves that's often the star of the show!), exploring the vaginal opening with gentle pressure, or inserting fingers into the vagina and using various motions like in-and-out movement or "come hither" curling to find the G-spot.

Pro tip: The clitoris has about 8,000 nerve endings and extends far beyond the little nub you can see. It actually looks more like a wishbone and encircles the vagina under the skin. Many people with vulvas need clitoral stimulation to experience orgasm. Lubricant is your friend here. Things feel better when they're slippery! Wash your hands beforehand and keep nails trimmed and smooth to prevent discomfort or tiny cuts.

Hand-to-Penis Play

Often called a handjob, hand job, or manual stimulation, this involves wrapping your hand(s) around the penis and moving up and down the shaft, paying special attention to the frenulum (that sensitive spot where the head meets the shaft on the underside), varying speed, pressure, and grip based on feedback, and sometimes including the testicles with gentle cupping or stroking.

Pro tip: Dry friction isn't usually pleasant, so use lube, lotion, or other slippery substances meant for sexual play. Communication is key—what works for one person might not work for another. A simple "Do you like this?" or telling the giver, "Faster or slower" can make all the difference.

Mutual Manual Play

This means partners manually stimulating each other simultaneously. It's a great way to learn what your partner enjoys while also receiving pleasure yourself.

There is a variation of Mutual Masturbation which involved each partner stimulating their own self while watching their partner/s do the same. This allows partners to see what each other likes as well as demonstrate what they like themselves.

Oral Sex: Using Your Mouth
Mouth-to-Vulva Play

Commonly called cunnilingus, going down, eating out, or giving head, this involves using your tongue to lick and stimulate the vulva, particularly the clitoris, potentially sucking gently on the clitoris or labia, sometimes including fingers for internal stimulation, and creating patterns with your tongue like circles, up-and-down, or side-to-side movements. Kissing or making out with a vulva can feel incredible and is a great place to start.

Pro tip: Consistency is often more important than fancy moves. Finding a rhythm and sticking with it, especially when your partner is approaching orgasm, can be more effective than constantly switching techniques. Dental dams can reduce STI transmission risk while still allowing for plenty of pleasure.

Mouth-to-Penis Play

Usually called fellatio, blow jobs, or giving head (yep, same term as above), this involves taking the penis into your mouth and creating suction and movement, using your tongue along the shaft and head, potentially including your hands to stimulate parts your mouth isn't covering, and varying depth, pressure, and speed.

Pro tip: Despite the term "blow job," it's not about blowing air—it's about suction and movement. And contrary to what porn might suggest, most people can't (and don't need to) take an entire penis into their throat. Condoms can be used for safer oral sex, with flavored options available for those who prefer them.

Mouth-to-Anus Play

Called rimming, analingus, or a rim job, this involves using your tongue to stimulate the anal opening, potentially inserting the tongue slightly, and sometimes combining with manual stimulation of genitals.

Pro tip: This area has lots of nerve endings and can be quite sensitive. Extra attention to hygiene is important, and dental dams are strongly recommended as barriers for safer sex. This activity carries higher risks for certain STIs without protection, so communication about testing and boundaries is especially important. This area also requires preparation and cleanliness to avoid bacterial infections.

Penetrative Sex: Putting Things Inside Other Things
Penis-in-Vagina Sex (PIV)

Often just called "sex" (though that's limiting!), this involves insertion of a penis into a vagina, movement that creates friction and stimulation for both partners, and various positions that change angles, depth, and control.

Pro tip: Most people with vaginas don't orgasm from penetration alone. Adding clitoral stimulation (with hands, toys, or positioning) can make a world of difference! Condoms are highly effective at preventing both pregnancy and STIs when used consistently and correctly.

Penis-in-Anus Sex (Anal)

Called anal sex or anal intercourse, this involves insertion of a penis into another person's anus, careful preparation including relaxation and lubrication, and gradual, patient penetration and movement.

Pro tip: The anus doesn't self-lubricate like a vagina, so lube is absolutely essential. Start slow, communicate constantly, and remember that discomfort is a sign to slow down or stop. Pain is never "just part of it." Condoms are crucial for safer anal sex, and changing condoms when switching between anal and other forms of penetration prevents harmful bacteria transfer.

Finger-in-Anus Play

Sometimes called fingering or digital penetration, this can be a sexual activity on its own, preparation for other types of anal play, or combined with other stimulation.

Pro tip: Start with one well-lubricated finger and make sure nails are trimmed and smooth. The rectum is only a few inches long and carries all the nerves, so deep penetration isn't necessary to hit pleasurable spots. Gloves can make cleanup easier and provide an additional barrier for safety.

Toy Penetration

Using specially designed sex toys for penetration of the vagina or anus includes dildos (non-vibrating penis-shaped or phallic objects), vibrators (electronic devices that vibrate for added stimulation), plugs (especially for anal play, with flared bases for safety), and strap-ons (dildos worn in a harness for partner penetration).

Pro tip: Always use toys designed for their intended purposes, especially for anal play, where toys **MUST** have a flared base to prevent them from getting lost inside. Different materials require different care and cleaning. Cover toys with condoms for easier cleanup and when sharing between partners.

Whole-Body Contact: Beyond the Genitals

Dry Humping / Outercourse

Rubbing bodies together, typically clothed or partially clothed, involves pressing genitals against a partner's body (thigh, hip, etc.), creating friction and pressure without penetration, and is often part of a sexual encounter but can be a complete sexual experience.

Pro tip: This often-overlooked activity can be extremely pleasurable and is a great option for safer sex or when penetration isn't desired. It's also perfect for exploring touch and pleasure with newer partners while maintaining boundaries.

Body-to-Genital Stimulation

Using non-genital body parts to stimulate genitals includes rubbing a penis between breasts (sometimes called "boob job"), stimulating genitals with feet ("foot job"), and rubbing genitals against various body parts.

Pro tip: These activities can add variety to your sexual repertoire and may be especially useful when dealing with certain physical limitations or preferences. They're also generally lower-risk activities for STI transmission.

Mutual Genital Rubbing

Direct contact between partners' genitals without penetration includes vulva-to-vulva contact (sometimes called "tribbing" or "scissoring"), penis-to-penis friction (sometimes called "frotting"), and vulva-to-penis external rubbing.

Pro tip: These activities can be plenty pleasurable on their own and also work as safer sex options with lower STI transmission risk than penetrative sex. Adding lubricant can enhance sensation and prevent uncomfortable friction.

Additional Intimate Activities

Kissing

From gentle pecks to deep tongue kissing, mouth-to-mouth contact is often a fundamental part of sexual interactions.

Pro tip: The lips are packed with nerve endings, making kissing intensely pleasurable all on its own. Pay attention to your partner's style and preferences, some like gentleness, others more passionate. Don't forget that kissing can involve tongues and gentle use of teeth. Start with gentle licks and light nips rather than aggressive techniques, you can always build intensity based on your partner's response. Kissing is like dancing, you're responding to how your partner responds. If they match and/or increase your action, keep going; if they retract or maintain their current action, dial down.

Erotic Massage

Using hands to rub, knead, and stroke non-genital body parts for pleasure can be a prelude to other sexual activities, may involve oils or lotions, and focuses on pleasure rather than therapeutic muscle work.

Pro tip: Take your time. A slow buildup creates anticipation and heightens sensitivity. Check in with your partner, asking things like "here?" "like this?" "how does that feel?" to find their sweet spot.

Nipple Play

Stimulating the nipples through touching, licking, sucking, or light pinching is something that all bodies can enjoy regardless of gender. Some people can even orgasm from nipple stimulation alone, and it can involve various intensities from gentle to more firm.

Pro tip: Nipple sensitivity varies enormously from person to person. Some love intense stimulation while others prefer gentle touch or even no direct contact. Start gentle and increase intensity only with positive feedback.

In Conclusion

This guide just scratches the surface of human sexual expression. Whatever activities you explore, remember these fundamentals: enthusiastic consent is non-negotiable, communication before, during, and after makes everything better, safer sex practices appropriate to the activity keep everyone healthy, personal boundaries deserve respect, and pleasure is the point. If it doesn't feel good, try something else!

There's no "right way" to have sex, just the way that works for you and your partner(s). Explore, communicate, be safe, and have fun!

Self-Pleasure: Masturbation, Baby!

Let's talk about masturbation. Seriously. How can you explain to someone else what gets you off if you don't know yourself? Self-pleasure isn't just some backup plan for when partners aren't available, it's a fundamental aspect of sexual wellness that deserves attention and respect.

The need for sexual pleasure is nearly universal. Even many asexually oriented persons still masturbate (though not all), because physical pleasure and sexual orientation are different aspects of human sexuality.

Why Self-Pleasure Matters

Self-knowledge is sexual power. When you know exactly how your body responds to different types of touch, pressure, and rhythm, you can communicate these preferences to partners. This isn't selfish, it's actually considerate. You're giving your partners the roadmap to pleasing you instead of making them guess.

It's yours alone. Sometimes it's genuinely refreshing not having to attend to another person's needs. Masturbation gives you complete freedom to focus entirely on your own pleasure without worrying about performance or someone else's enjoyment. It's one of the few sexual experiences that can be entirely about you.

Health benefits are real. Masturbation releases tension, improves sleep quality, reduces stress, and can even help with menstrual cramps or headaches for some people. It triggers the release of endorphins and dopamine—natural mood elevators that can help combat depression and anxiety.

It can enhance partnered sex. Contrary to outdated beliefs, regular masturbation doesn't diminish partnered experiences. It often enhances them. You're maintaining your sexual response system and staying connected to your desires.

Masturbation doesn't have to stop when you're in a relationship. In fact, it can become an exciting element of your partnered sex life:

Mutual masturbation can be incredibly intimate and arousing. Watching how your partner touches themselves provides valuable information about what they enjoy while also creating a vulnerable, trust-building experience.

Masturbation as foreplay can build anticipation and arousal before partnered activities. Starting with self-touch and then transitioning to partner touch creates a natural progression of escalating pleasure. And it's hot as fuck to watch someone touch themselves and see how excited they are.

Sometimes it's just practical. Different sex drives, physical distance, or temporary physical limitations don't have to mean sexual frustration. Self-pleasure helps bridge these gaps while maintaining sexual wellness.

Beyond Basic Techniques

There's a lot more to masturbation than the basics. Exploring different approaches can lead to more intense pleasure and new discoveries about your body:

For penis owners: Experiment with different strokes, pressures, and rhythms. There are specialized toys like strokers, sleeves, and vibrating rings designed specifically for penises that create sensations impossible to achieve by hand. Adding anal stimulation through prostate massage can dramatically intensify orgasms—this isn't about sexual orientation, it's about anatomy. The male equivalent of the g spot is the prostate, it sits about an inch inside your rectum and when its rubbed creates an ecstatic feeling. But you can only get there through the asshole…

For vagina owners: The clitoris has approximately 8,000 nerve endings and extends far beyond the visible nub. In fact, it extends down the sides of the vulva as well as internally. Explore different types of touch, direct or indirect, circles or tapping, varying pressure. Internal stimulation of the G-spot (located about 1-3 inches inside the vagina on the front wall) often produces different sensations from external stimulation. Combining these through toys or techniques can lead to blended orgasms of remarkable intensity.

For everyone: Experiment with temperature; warm or cool, (frozen dildo anyone?), different textures, vibration at various intensities, and edging (bringing yourself close to orgasm repeatedly before finally allowing release). Using lubricant, even if you don't think you need it, can significantly enhance sensations.

Getting Started with Toys

Sex toys aren't just for people who are "kinky" or "can't get the real thing." They're tools that can provide sensations no human hand or body part can replicate:

Vibrators come in countless forms, from tiny bullet vibes to wand massagers. They're not just for vaginas. They feel amazing on any erogenous zone.

Insertable toys designed for G-spot or prostate stimulation have curves and shapes specifically engineered to reach these pleasure points effectively.

Strokers and sleeves for penises create sensations of suction, texture, and pressure that hands simply can't replicate.

Anal toys (with proper flared bases for safety) can add entirely new dimensions to masturbation for all body types.

When selecting toys, look for body-safe materials like medical-grade silicone, borosilicate glass, or ABS plastic, and always clean them according to manufacturer instructions (usually just warm soapy water). Anything going in the butt needs to have a flared base, unless you like embarrassing trips to the ER.

Final Thoughts

Masturbation isn't just some consolation prize when "actual sex" isn't available. It's a valid, valuable sexual activity in its own right that deserves to be approached with curiosity, enthusiasm, and without shame. Whether you're single, partnered, or anything in between, getting to know your own body is one of the most empowering sexual skills you can develop.

So go ahead, make time for self-exploration. Your future self (and your partners) will thank you.

The Orgasm Trap: Why Chasing Climax Ruins Sex

"Did you cum?" is the worst fucking thing a guy can ask after sex.

This question (though often well-intentioned) immediately transforms what should have been a connected experience into a performance evaluation. It's like asking "did you win?" after dancing together. You missed the entire point.

The Problem with Goal-Oriented Sex

Obviously, we all want to orgasm. That intense pleasure is amazing, and for many, it feels like the natural conclusion to sexual activity. But here's the uncomfortable truth: fixating on orgasm is the fastest way to prevent it from happening.

When orgasm becomes the goal rather than a potential outcome, sex transforms from an exploratory, pleasure-focused experience into a task with a pass/fail grade. This creates pressure, and pressure is the ultimate boner killer, both literally and figuratively.

As much as it's nice to arrive every now and then; we're focused on the journey, not the destination.

What Porn Gets Wrong About Pleasure

Mainstream porn showcases a marathon sprint toward the money shot. Everything is performed with orgasm as the singular purpose and validation that the sex was "successful."

But porn is entertainment, not a documentary! Real sex rarely follows this linear path toward simultaneous, earth-shattering orgasms. In reality, arousal ebbs and flows. Sensations build and recede. Bodies don't always cooperate with our desires.

Great sex starts with showing up genuinely and enthusiastically. Not with a script or a checklist, but with curiosity about your partner's body and responses. After that, focus on a radical idea: making each other feel good in the present moment.

"Do you like this?"

"Would you prefer it harder?"

"Right there or move lower?"

And from the receiving end:

"Yes."

"Slower."

"Don't stop."

"A little to the left."

These simple exchanges create connection and amplify pleasure because they anchor both of you in the immediate experience rather than some future goal. They acknowledge that pleasure is happening right now, not just building toward something later.

The Psychology of Pleasure Problems

For many people, the pressure to orgasm (especially to make their partner feel skilled or validated) becomes an intrusive thought; and intrusive thoughts are orgasm assassins.

For all genders, but women especially, mental distractions can demolish arousal. Worries like "Am I taking too long?" or "Do I look weird from this angle?" start spiraling through your head. You're wondering "What if I can't finish?" or "Are they getting bored?" and suddenly you're completely out of the moment and stuck in your own anxious brain.

Most cases of anorgasmia (inability to reach orgasm) don't stem from physical issues but from psychological barriers; particularly these performance anxieties. Similarly, many men who experience erectile difficulties find that their equipment works perfectly fine until sex is on the table and the pressure to perform kicks in.

Women also commonly face the flawed expectation that penetrative sex alone should produce orgasm, when in reality, only about 18% of women reliably orgasm from penetration without additional clitoral stimulation.

A Better Approach to Sexual Pleasure

Instead of approaching sex with orgasm as the non-negotiable goal, try these mindset shifts:

1. **Redefine success**: Good sex is about connection, pleasure, and exploration, not a specific physical response.
2. **Stay present**: Focus on the sensation happening right now rather than what's supposed to happen next.
3. **Communicate without scorekeeping**: Feedback like "that feels amazing" is different from "I'm almost there," because it celebrates current pleasure rather than progress toward a goal. It should be noted that for penis owners, a warning that ejaculation is about to happen is often a polite courtesy, especially during oral sex.
4. **Remove time pressure**: Some of the best sexual experiences happen when there's no deadline or expected end point.
5. **Embrace variability**: Sometimes you'll orgasm quickly, sometimes after a long build-up, sometimes not at all; and that's completely normal.

Here's the ironic part: when you stop obsessively chasing orgasms, they often happen more easily. The lack of pressure to perform and reach some arbitrary finish line creates the mental freedom necessary for pleasure to build naturally.

Great sexual experiences aren't about checking boxes or reaching milestones. They're about being fully present with another human's body and your own, exploring what feels good without judgment or expectation.

So, the next time you're tempted to ask, "did you cum?" try these instead: "That was incredible," or "I love how your body responds when I..." or "What was your favorite part?" or "I'd love to try more of that thing that made you moan."

Because ultimately, great sex isn't about what happened at the end; it's about how connected, pleased, and present you felt throughout the entire experience.

CHAPTER THREE

Gender

The Standard Narrative: The Script That Was Given To You

The "Standard Narrative" is that invisible script running through our society that we all absorbed without realizing it needed questioning. It's the background noise defining what "normal" supposedly looks like.

You know it intimately: Men are like this; women are like that. People are born male or female, period. Relationships follow one predictable path - meet, date, marry, have kids, stay together forever. One man, one woman. Happily ever after.

This narrative isn't just some abstract concept - it's hardwired into everything from children's books to wedding ceremonies to medical forms. It's the default setting, the path of least resistance, the story we're all pressured to follow.

I get why this narrative is comforting. Clean categories and clear expectations provide a sense of order in a chaotic world. The problem is, they're bullshit.

Some people's stories do follow the standard narrative, just like some people are white. But that doesn't mean everyone is white or that everyone's relationships, genders, and orientations conform to this one script. Nature doesn't give a shit about our neat little categories. Human bodies, identities, and relationships are wildly more diverse than this one plot line allows. The Standard Narrative isn't reality; it's a cultural construction that's been around so long we mistake it for natural law.

This matters because when we treat a simplified model as the only acceptable reality, we cause real harm to real people. Those who don't fit the narrative aren't just different; they're made out to be the enemy. Ask any trans kid in a state banning their healthcare, or any polyamorous family fighting for legal recognition, or any intersex person who underwent unnecessary surgeries as an infant.

As someone who's spent years watching people struggle against these invisible boundaries, I'm convinced that understanding the Standard Narrative is vital to understanding each other. Some parts of it might fit for you, some parts won't and that's good.

What Does It Mean to Be Transgender?

At its core, being transgender means your sense of who you are doesn't match the gender everyone told you that you were based on your body parts at birth. It's that simple and that complex at the same time.

Think about it this way: Most people are born with certain physical characteristics, and society immediately says, "You're a boy" or "You're a girl" based on those characteristics. Most commonly it's the presence of a penis or vagina at birth. For cisgender people (non-transgender folks), this label feels right. Their internal sense of who they are aligns with what the doctor announced when they were born. No conflict there.

For transgender people, this isn't the case. There's a persistent, fundamental disconnect between their inner sense of gender and what is visible to society. It isn't about liking "boy things" or "girl things" plenty of masculine women and feminine men are perfectly comfortable with their assigned gender; and coming to terms with liking traditionally opposite gendered things is a different discussion. This is about a deeper identity that doesn't line up with social expectations.

This disconnect often creates distress called gender dysphoria - which can feel like wearing clothes that are completely the wrong size, except it's your body that feels wrong. It's like looking in a mirror and seeing a stranger staring back at you. Not every trans person experiences dysphoria the same way or to the same degree, but that fundamental mismatch is what ultimately defines the transgender experience.

Being transgender isn't a mental illness, a trend, or a choice. It's simply a natural variation in human experience. Trans people have existed in virtually every culture throughout human history, though different cultures have understood and labeled this experience in vastly different ways. In Native American cultures, for example, the term Two Spirit (in translation) identified people who didn't fit gender norms, and they were often revered as individuals who could walk two paths, experience multiple realities, and offer unique wisdom to their communities.

It's also worth noting that gender isn't always binary. While some trans people identify strongly as men or women, others experience their gender somewhere in between or outside these categories entirely. The umbrella term of transgender includes people who identify as a combination of both, as different genders at different times, or as something else entirely. Non-binary has emerged as its own recognized category for many whose gender doesn't fit neatly into male or female boxes.

The question of why some people are transgender doesn't have a single answer. Current research suggests a complex interplay of biological, psychological, and social factors. What's clear is that gender identity forms deep in our sense of self, typically by early childhood, and attempts to force someone to identify differently than they authentically feel can cause significant harm.

While being transgender and being intersex are distinct experiences, they both challenge the idea that sex and gender are simple binaries. Intersex conditions occur when a person's physical development doesn't follow typical male or female patterns. There are approximately 40 variations affecting chromosomes, hormones, or anatomical development. Most intersex people are assigned a gender at birth, but like anyone else, that assignment may not match their eventual gender identity.

Understanding transgender experiences means recognizing that the simple categories we're taught as children don't capture the full spectrum of human diversity. When we listen to people telling us who they are rather than assuming based on appearance, we move toward a world where everyone can live authentically.

Beyond the Regret Narrative: Understanding Gender Transition in Context

The debate around gender-affirming care often fixates on a single narrative: young people making irreversible decisions they'll later regret. This concern, while emotionally compelling to many parents and policymakers, deserves a more nuanced examination than it typically receives.

Let's acknowledge reality first: detransition does happen. Recent peer-reviewed studies estimate that roughly 1-4% of people who pursue medical transition later reverse course. However, these statistics require context that's frequently missing from public discourse.

When we examine cases of detransition more carefully, several patterns emerge:

First, the timing matters. Genuine gender dysphoria typically has a persistent, consistent history stretching back years, often to early childhood. Cases where someone suddenly identifies as transgender during adolescence without previous gender incongruence may indeed warrant a more measured approach to medical interventions. This isn't about denying identity but ensuring appropriate care.

Second, social factors do influence gender exploration. Humans are social creatures. We all seek community and belonging. Some young people may initially be drawn to trans communities for acceptance, particularly if they're struggling with other aspects of identity or mental health. However, this doesn't mean their gender identity is "fake" or that gender-affirming care should be withheld. It means mental health professionals should explore multiple factors contributing to distress.

What's missing from simplistic "they'll regret it" arguments is an understanding of how gender-affirming care actually works in practice:

1. Social transition (changing names, pronouns, presentation) carries no medical risk and is fully reversible
2. Puberty blockers are reversible interventions that create time for exploration
3. Hormone therapy produces some irreversible changes, which is why it requires more thorough evaluation
4. Surgical interventions for minors are exceedingly rare and

typically limited to older teens after years of consistent gender identity

The conversation around transition regret also fails to acknowledge an uncomfortable truth: denying care to transgender youth carries its own significant risks, including depression, anxiety, and suicide. Any honest risk assessment must weigh potential regret against these documented harms.

Ultimately, the most ethical approach isn't blanket approval or denial of care, but individualized assessment by qualified professionals who can distinguish between different pathways to gender incongruence and recommend appropriate, staged interventions based on each person's unique situation.

Gender Benders: Understanding Gender Expression and Identity

Gender expression comes in many forms beyond the simple male/female binary we're often taught. To build a more inclusive understanding, it helps to explore the nuances of how people express their gender through clothing, behavior, and identity. Let's break down some terms that often get confused or misunderstood.

Crossdressers

Crossdressing is simply wearing clothing typically associated with another gender. This is the broadest term here, covering a wide range of motivations and experiences. Some people crossdress for personal comfort, some for sexual pleasure, some for performance, and some as an expression of gender identity.

The crucial thing to understand is that crossdressing says nothing definitive about someone's sexual orientation or gender identity - straight cisgender men, gay cisgender men, and people across the gender and sexuality spectrum may crossdress. For many, it's about the freedom to express different aspects of themselves rather than a statement about who they fundamentally are. An example is drag queens. Often drag queens identify as men but dress up in exaggeratedly feminine costume and star in shows (or readings) as performance art. RuPaul is an example. Queens are often part of the queer community but not necessarily transgender.

Transvestites

"Transvestite" is largely an outdated clinical term that was once used to describe crossdressers. It has fallen out of favor because of its pathologizing history and clinical connotations that treated gender-nonconforming behavior as a disorder.

Many people who might have been labeled this way in the past would now use terms like "crossdresser" instead. In some contexts, particularly in older communities or in certain European countries, some people still identify with this term, but it's generally not used in contemporary discussions unless someone specifically identifies that way.

Femboys

Femboys (sometimes written as "fembois") generally refers to people who were assigned male at birth who present in ways that are feminine but still identify as male or masculine in some capacity. The aesthetic often involves a youthful, androgynous appearance incorporating feminine clothing, makeup, and mannerisms while retaining some masculine elements.

The term has gained popularity in online communities and can represent both a fashion aesthetic and a gender expression. For some, it's purely about style; for others, it reflects a more complex gender identity. Like many contemporary gender terms, "femboy" has evolved rapidly and carries different meanings in different communities.

Sissy

"Sissy" exists in several contexts. It originated as a derogatory term for effeminate men but has been reclaimed in certain communities. In BDSM and fetish contexts, "sissy" often refers to a specific form of role-play or identity that eroticizes feminization, often with elements of humiliation or power exchange.

Outside sexual contexts, some people use it as an identity label that embraces a particular form of femininity. Because of its complicated history and potential to be used as a slur, it's a term that should generally only be used by or for people who explicitly identify with it.

Important Distinctions

The key thing to understand is that these are all forms of gender expression, not necessarily gender identity. Most (though not all) people in these categories don't consider themselves transgender in the sense of having a gender identity that differs from their assigned sex at birth. For many, these expressions are about exploring gender presentation without changing gender identity.

That said, for some people, these forms of expression can be part of a journey of gender exploration that might eventually lead to identifying as transgender or non-binary. Others may find that these forms of expression satisfy their needs to express gender in ways that differ from societal expectations, without necessarily changing how they identify.

Many of these communities have developed their own rich histories, cultural touchstones, and support networks over decades, showing how gender expression has always been more diverse than mainstream society acknowledges.

There's no hierarchy here. These are just different ways people express and explore gender; and each deserves respect as a valid form of self-expression. Understanding these distinctions helps us move past judgment and toward appreciating the full spectrum of how humans experience and express gender.

CHAPTER FOUR

Orientation

Are You Gay?: Why Labels Don't Tell the Whole Story

We typically think if someone of one binary gender is attracted to people of the same binary gender, they're "gay," right? But the relationship between sexual identity and sexual behavior is far more complex than our labels suggest.

Let's consider what we mean by "identity" in the first place. How a person identifies is essentially how they present themselves to the outside world. The phrase "I identify as..." has become common in our cultural language because identity serves as a social function. These labels (straight, gay, bi, heteroflexible, pan) primarily exist to communicate something about ourselves to others. In the privacy of our own thoughts, what matters is simply what we desire, not what we call it. The label is for others.

This distinction between identity and behavior becomes particularly evident when we look at straight-identifying men who have sex with other men. These individuals don't identify as gay or bisexual and often maintain long-term relationships with women, yet occasionally (or regularly) engage in sexual activities with men. Their straight identity remains intact because that's how they understand themselves and how they wish to be seen by the world.

There are numerous reasons why a straight-identifying person might engage in same-sex activities. They might be predominantly attracted to the opposite gender but occasionally experience same-sex attraction, or they might enjoy stepping outside their usual sexual role for the novelty or taboo aspect. The behavior might be situational, as in environments where opposite-sex partners aren't available, or they might simply enjoy certain sexual activities regardless of who's providing them. It could be a specific kink that doesn't align with their overall sexual orientation, or they might enjoy the secrecy or transgressive nature of the experience. They might also not want to change their entire social identity for something that represents only a portion of their sexuality.

It's tempting to dismiss these individuals as "just closeted" or "in denial," but that perspective oversimplifies human sexuality. Most aspects of sexuality exist on a spectrum rather than in neat either/or categories. A straight-identifying man might genuinely be predominantly attracted to women, desire a conventional heterosexual relationship, and only occasionally enjoy same-sex encounters.

Our culture's standard narrative associates certain behaviors exclusively with specific identities, i.e. if you engage in same-sex behavior, you must be gay or bisexual. This creates a problem for people whose behaviors and identities don't align with these expectations. For many straight-identifying men, "gay" carries negative connotations within their social circles, making them resistant to that label regardless of their behaviors. And bisexual comes with its own set of judgments, both inside and out of the gay community.

This disconnection between identity and behavior isn't limited to men, though women's experiences often manifest differently due to different social pressures and expectations. Women who engage in same-sex behavior while identifying as straight are often viewed through a different cultural lens; sometimes dismissed as "just experimenting" or "performing" for male attention rather than expressing authentic desire. This is common in the swinging community (aka lifestyle community) where couple swapping often starts with the women engaging with each other regardless of their actual orientation. Additionally, it is more socially acceptable for women to express affection to other women physically than it is for men to express similar affection physically. Girls can hold hands as "besties" and still be considered straight, whereas men holding hands is exclusively gay.

Understanding the distinction between identity and behavior helps us recognize that sexual orientation is more complex than simple labels suggest. People choose the identities that best represent their overall sense of self, even when their behaviors might sometimes suggest different categories to outside observers. Respecting how people identify and choose to express themselves, while acknowledging the complexity of human sexuality, creates space for more honest conversations about desire and deeper opportunities for authentic connection.

Understanding LGBTQ+ Identities

The term "queer community" has become common shorthand for people whose sexuality or gender identity doesn't fit the standard straight/cisgender narrative. "Queer" was historically used as a slur against anyone with same-gender attractions, but it's been reclaimed by the LGBTQ+ community. However, straight people should still be careful using it, as it can still function as a slur depending on context and intent.

Let's break down what the letters actually mean:

L = Lesbian: Women who are sexually and romantically attracted to other women.

G = Gay: Men who are sexually and romantically attracted to other men. (Sometimes used as an umbrella term for all same-gender attractions.)

B = Bisexual: People attracted to both their own gender and other genders. This can include attraction to men and women, or a broader range of gender identities.

T = Transgender: Here's where we shift gears. The first three letters describe sexual orientation - who you're attracted to. Transgender refers to gender identity - how you understand your own gender. Trans people are those whose gender identity differs from what was assigned at birth. This is completely separate from sexual orientation - trans people can be straight, gay, bisexual, or any other orientation.

Q = Queer or Questioning: This serves as both a catch-all umbrella term and a specific identity. As an umbrella, "queer" can include anyone whose sexuality or gender doesn't fit standard narrative. As "questioning," it refers to people exploring aspects of their sexuality &/or gender identity. There's no set timeline or required process for questioning. It's not a one-time decision you make at 16 and stick with forever. For many people, their sense of sexuality and gender evolve throughout their lives.

Important note: These definitions continue to evolve, and people within LGBTQ+ communities sometimes disagree on terminology. What matters most is respecting how individuals identify themselves.

Coming Out: The Universal Experience of Authenticity

"Coming out" originally meant "coming out of the closet" - when someone reveals their sexual orientation or gender identity after keeping it private. But here's the thing: coming out isn't just about being LGBTQ+.

Coming out happens anytime your internal sense of self doesn't match what your community expects, and you decide to stop pretending. It can be about sexual orientation, gender identity, kink preferences, relationship styles like ENM, or even philosophical beliefs. Liberal in a conservative family? Atheist in a religious community? Those are coming-out moments too.

I've had two major coming-out experiences: 1st; telling my Christian family and friends I don't actually believe in God anymore. 2nd: Having to tell my parents, who were coming to visit, that my girlfriend was living with me and my wife. Both required the same courage to say "this is who I really am."

For people with supportive communities, coming out might be a rite of passage that surprises no one. But for most people, it involves real risk; rejection by family, friends, &/or community. Sometimes this rejection escalates to physical violence. There are communities that preach love and peace but only for their own members, practicing hate and violence against outsiders. Many LGBTQ+ people have been kicked out of their families simply for existing.

Because of these real consequences, coming out is deeply personal. Never pressure someone else to come out; you don't know what they're risking. Physical safety, financial stability, and emotional support can all be on the line.

But when it is safe enough to come out, most people experience profound relief. There's peace in having your internal sense of self align with how you present to the world.

Coming out isn't a one-time event; it's something people navigate throughout their lives in different contexts. Being out at work doesn't automatically mean being out with family. Being out with friends doesn't mean being out everywhere else. Each situation requires its own calculation of safety versus authenticity.

This is why coming out deserves respect, support, and patience. Whether it's about sexuality, gender, beliefs, or any other fundamental part of who someone is.

CHAPTER FIVE

Flirting

The Art of Flirting: A Positive-Sum Game

Flirting is expressing interest in someone but doing it in a playful way that invites them to respond to your advances. It's a game; but not the kind where someone has to lose.

When frat boys or fuckboys talk about "having game," they're operating in a zero-sum mindset: they win, the other person loses. Fuck that.

Real flirting is a positive-sum game, where both people win by having a genuinely good time, regardless of where things end up. Flirting is about the journey, not the destination.

Flirting is fundamentally about having fun. If you're just trying to get laid, there are more direct ways to achieve that goal without the manipulative bullshit. Using flirting (or anything else) as a way to trick someone into fucking you makes you an asshole, plain and simple. Don't be a dick. The reason flirting is a game is that games are fun; and games are the most fun when all the people playing know they're playing.

What makes flirting exciting? It's an unspoken understanding. It's that electric current running between you both that neither person explicitly names. It's like sharing a secret without saying a word. Example:

You: "I've been told I make a killer margarita."
Them: "Oh really? I'd have to verify that claim personally."
You: "I guess you would. For scientific purposes, of course."

Them: "Purely scientific. I take my research very seriously."

Neither person directly said, "Let's have drinks at your place," but you both know exactly what's being discussed.

Read the Room (Seriously)

Not everyone gets off on ambiguity. Some folks, including many on the neurodivergent spectrum, but plenty of others too, prefer clarity over hints. Flirting effectively means adapting to how the other person communicates.

Watch how they respond to your initial flirts: Do they lean in and match your energy? Do they seem confused or uncomfortable? Are they flirting back but in a different style?

The best flirts are adaptable and can switch up their approach based on what works for their partner. Some people prefer witty banter, others respond to sincere compliments, some want direct statements of interest with clear intentions, and some want to be pursued. Figure out what style the other person likes and use that. Or, if you're not into that style, totally fine! It's not a match, politely move on.

Handle Rejection Like a Grown-Up

Rejection is not an insult, unless you've been being a dick, then you deserve the insult. But someone communicating to you that they're not interested is a kindness! It saves you time and energy that you can put to better use elsewhere.

Also, it's not necessarily personal. If they aren't into you, that doesn't mean there's something wrong with you. It means you're not their particular flavor, and that's okay; you're someone else's perfect taste. If they aren't into you, someone else will be.

When you get rejected: Thank them (internally or externally) for being clear. Then exit gracefully without making it weird. Remember: their "no" has saved you from wasting time on a dead end

Playing Hard to Get (Advanced Mode)

When done right, this dynamic can be hot as fuck for both parties. Some people enjoy the chase, others enjoy being pursued. When these two types connect—fireworks.

But this is where shit gets complicated. How do you tell the difference between someone playing hard to get and someone who's genuinely not interested?

As the chaser you have to pay attention to the kind of running your "prey" is making. There should be playfulness evident in their responses. There might be deflections, retorts, sarcasm and humor that are freely thrown around, but there isn't a solid "no thank you," "go away," "I'm not interested," or other versions of disinterest.

Signals to Watch For:

"Maybe" signals (green light to continue flirting):

They deflect direct advances but stay engaged in conversation

You: "Can I get your number?"

Them: "I barely know you yet! Where are you from?" (while smiling and continuing the conversation rather than shutting it down)

They use playful sarcasm or teasing

You: "I'm actually a pretty good cook."

Them: "Oh really? Is microwaving ramen your specialty?" (challenging you in a playful way that invites response) tone and body language matter here.

Their body language remains open and attentive

They maintain eye contact, face their body toward you, play with their hair, or find small excuses to decrease physical distance (like leaning in to hear you better even when it's not that loud)

They might say "I don't normally do this, but..." (creating token resistance while actually showing interest)

"I don't usually talk to strangers at bars, but you seem interesting." "I should probably get back to my friends, but I'm enjoying our conversation too much."

"No" signals (time to back off):

They give short, closed responses

You: "What kind of music are you into?"

Them: "Different stuff." (no elaboration, no follow-up question)

They physically turn away or increase distance

They position their body toward the exit or their friends instead of you. They take a step back when you step forward. They cross their arms or create barriers with objects (holding their drink up between you).

They mention partners or lack of interest in dating

"My boyfriend/girlfriend and I just watched that movie..." "I'm really focusing on myself right now, not looking to date anyone." "I'm just out with friends tonight, not looking to meet anyone."

They directly say "I'm not interested" or "No thanks"

You: "Could I buy you a drink?"

Them: "No thanks, I'm good." (without offering an alternative)

As the person being chased (and liking it), your role in the game is to incite the chaser to keep chasing. It's like a game of tag where you want to be caught. You can't run too fast because you'll actually escape, you can't run too slow because you'll be caught too soon. Your job is sending clear "maybes" not firm "nos."

If you're actually not interested send clear "no's."

Digital Flirting: The Text Game

Flirting via text or dating apps comes with its own set of signals and challenges. Without body language to guide you, pay closer attention to these cues:

Maybe signals in digital spaces include quick, consistent responses and messages that end with questions to keep the conversation going. They might use emojis, GIFs, or memes that match your energy, or suggest moving to another platform like going from a dating app to exchanging phone numbers or from texting to video calls.

No signals in digital spaces show up as long delays between responses and one-word answers with no follow-ups. They only respond to direct questions without ever initiating conversation themselves, and repeatedly avoid suggestions to meet or talk outside the app.

Digital flirting tip: When in doubt, be slightly more direct than you would in person. Text lacks tone, so playfulness can sometimes be read as disinterest.

Consent Is Non-Negotiable

"Your mouth says no but your eyes say yes" is NOT consent for physical contact. Eye contact, smiles, and flirtatious banter give you permission to continue the verbal dance; not to touch.

Physical escalation requires clearer signals: They initiate touch (hand on arm, shoulder bump). They verbally invite closer contact ("Want to sit somewhere quieter?"). They respond positively when you ask ("Would it be okay if I moved a little closer?")

Safety First, Always

Protect yourself when flirting with strangers, or when strangers are flirting with you: Notice how other people respond to this person.

Are people moving away from them? Not laughing at their jokes? Check in with friends about the vibe they're getting. Ask yourself: What might they want beyond my charming personality?

Pay attention to your environment as well. If you're a man approaching a woman in an alley or deserted street, not the best place for flirtations. That's fucking scary dude.

If you're approaching someone new, respect their initial caution. It's not a personal insult if someone's guard is up; that's just smart self-preservation. If they're clearly not interested, move on gracefully. It's probably not about you, until you act like a dickhead and make it about you. Don't be that asshole who makes it weird.

The Exit Strategy

Sometimes you start flirting and realize—nope, not feeling it. That's completely fine. You can always politely exit:

"It's been great talking with you, but I should get back to my friends. " Or, "I need to head out, but it was nice meeting you."

Simple, direct, and not a dick move.

Recovering from Missteps

We all fuck up sometimes. Maybe you misread a signal, made someone uncomfortable, or came on too strong. How you recover matters more than the mistake:

1. **Acknowledge it briefly**: "Sorry, I misread that situation."
2. **Don't over-explain or make it worse**: No need for a lengthy apology, that makes things more awkward
3. **Give them space**: Back off physically and conversationally
4. **Move on gracefully**: Change the subject or make your exit

The difference between being weird and being someone who just made a mistake is how you handle it afterward.

Breaking the Fourth Wall (Rare but Useful)

Occasionally, explicitly naming what's happening can be powerful:

"Just so we're clear—I'm flirting with you right now."

"I'm enjoying this back-and-forth we have going."

This works especially well with people who appreciate directness or when there's potential for misunderstanding.

A Note on Cultural Differences

Flirting varies across cultures. What reads as forward in one context might be considered tame in another. When flirting across cultural backgrounds: Pay extra attention to how your advances are received. Be more specific if there seems to be confusion. Respect that comfort levels with directness vary widely around the world

Flirting should leave both people feeling good regardless of how far it goes or where it ends up. If it led to more fun in the physical sense, great! But remember just trying to get laid is usually pretty obvious and if that's not what the other person wants, you're more likely to come off as creepy than charming.

Even if it was just a fun interaction that went nowhere, if it brought a smile or laugh to yours and their faces or boosted yours or their confidence or ego, that's a fucking win! Or if it just helped you figure out you weren't compatible, consider it practice. However it goes, if someone walks away feeling manipulated or disrespected, you're doing it wrong.

The real masters of flirting aren't the ones who "score" the most. They're the ones who create enjoyable experiences regardless of the outcome.

Teasing vs. Negging: Know the Fucking Difference

The key feature of good teasing is that it's not "negging." Negging is when some fuckboi uses actual insults to trigger a reverse psychology response in their target. I say target because negging is fundamentally manipulative. It's fucked up to insult people, and it's fucked up to try to trick people into sex through emotional manipulation.

Real teasing is playful. The person being teased should know they're being flirted with and should walk away feeling good about themselves, not insulted or diminished. This comes down to tone and body language more than your actual words. The goal is to gently poke fun while simultaneously signaling that the thing you're teasing about is actually something you find endearing or attractive about them.

Here's the thing: the whole point of flirting is to show someone you like them. It's a playful game with two purposes. First, to indicate you're interested. Second, to find out if they might be interested back.

Good teasing guidelines: Punch up or sideways, never down at insecurities or things they can't control. Include yourself in the joke sometimes; this shows you're not putting yourself above them. Balance it with genuine compliments. If they seem uncomfortable or don't respond well, back off immediately.

Remember: if someone feels worse about themselves after your "teasing," you've crossed into asshole territory. The litmus test is simple. Would they tell their friends about your interaction with a smile or a grimace?

Don't overuse teasing either. It's like seasoning, a little goes a long way. Too much and you just sound like you're constantly making fun of them, which defeats the whole purpose of showing you're interested.

Compliments: Your Gateway Drug to Better Social Skills

Everyone likes being complimented, and here's the beautiful thing, it's a skill you can practice without any flirting pressure. Shy? Not around anyone you're interested in? It doesn't matter. You can still sharpen this tool. Bonus: giving genuine compliments is a mood booster when you're having a shit day. Making someone else feel good makes you feel good. Try simply smiling kindly (not creepily) at people you pass.

The formula is dead simple: Pick a feature that's not too personal or body-focused, like shoes, nails, clothing, hair and say, "I like your ____." That's it. They'll say, "thank you" and either stay quiet or try small talk. Small talk is where you can start testing the flirting waters.

Real-world example: At work in a jail setting, a nurse is sitting by the window watching inmates play volleyball in the yard.

Man: "I like your shoes." Nurse: "Thanks." [looks shyly toward the yard] "I've never seen them play volleyball before. Usually it's basketball." Man: "I know, right? What's next, knitting?" Nurse: [chuckles politely].

Let's be honest, that joke isn't hilarious. But that's not the point. The point is reading her response. She gave a polite chuckle, which signals "you can continue this interaction." If she'd gone silent or given a flat "huh," that would mean "I'm not interested in talking to you."

Here's the crucial part: Her chuckle doesn't mean she's definitely interested in you romantically. It just means she's open to finding out what this interaction is about. She might not even realize flirting is happening yet.

Reading the signals:

Green lights: Smiles, sustained eye contact, playing with hair, open body language, giggling, asking questions back.

Yellow lights: Polite responses, brief answers, looking away occasionally.

Red lights: One-word answers, closed body language, checking phone, looking for escape routes.

The intensity rule: Generally, more animated responses mean more interest. But if someone's being more animated about saying "no" or "stop" then that intensity means LESS interest. Read the fucking room.

Critical warning: "Maybe" or yellow light responses usually mean "no, but I'm being polite." Don't mistake politeness for invitation. When someone's genuinely interested, they'll start sending flirts back and more than once. That's when you know you've got a willing participant in the game. Getting one "maybe" response doesn't mean quit, getting a few "maybe's" means move on.

Don't be the person who remembers every tiny interaction and builds it into something bigger. If you're thinking 'but she smiled at me three weeks ago,' and you see her every day, you're already in fantasy land. If you must reach back weeks for your "evidence" that someone's interested, that's your answer right there.

The whole point is paying attention to how your compliments land and adjust accordingly. People don't always respond perfectly in the moment, but persistent disinterest is a clear message. Don't be willfully ignorant of someone's decline to play.

Sarcasm: Your Humor Filter (Use Carefully)

I've noticed that when I use sarcasm *at* someone it tends to be received as an insult. Unless we're already friends. Whereas when I use sarcasm *next* to someone it simply says something about yourself that they can decide if they want to know more about.

Picture this: you're in a group with friends, and you make a sarcastic joke that gets some people laughing and others looking uncomfortable. Boom! You've just identified who might be open to your style of flirting and who definitely isn't. It's like a humor compatibility test that saves everyone time and awkwardness.

The problem: There's a razor-thin line between playful sarcasm and asshole sarcasm, especially from the recipient's perspective. It's easy as fuck to accidentally come across as mean when you think you're being funny.

The safer approach: Self-deprecating sarcasm. When you're the target of your own joke, you're showing you can laugh at yourself without putting anyone else down. It's disarming and often attractive because it signals confidence, humor, and humility at the same time.

Here's some examples:

Risky: "Wow, someone's really dressed to impress today" (sarcasm AT someone about their outfit)

Safer: "And here I am looking like I got dressed in the dark again" (sarcasm about your own outfit, NEXT TO others)

Risky: "Oh, you're one of those people who gets up at 5am to work out" (sarcasm AT their habits)

Safer: "Meanwhile, I consider it a workout when I have to walk upstairs to get my phone charger" (sarcasm about your own laziness, NEXT TO others)

The pattern is always the same: instead of making them the punchline, make yourself the punchline while everyone else gets to enjoy the joke.

Targeting insecurities or things people can't control is where sarcasm can cross the line. So is punching down at someone's genuine enthusiasm; a total dick move. Using it before you've built any rapport is unwise. And read the room; some groups/cultures don't do sarcasm.

Remember, sarcasm is a spice, not the main dish. Use it to show your personality, not to tear others down. If people consistently don't laugh at your sarcastic jokes, that's valuable information about either your delivery or your audience. Pay attention and adjust accordingly.

Touch and Consent in U.S. Culture

In US culture, touch is a big fucking deal. We don't just go around touching people. There's a whole social dance around it. Even something as basic as a handshake involves an offer (extending your hand) that the other person can accept or politely dodge.

Most Americans are pretty touch-conservative with people they don't know well. Hugs with strangers? That's usually reserved for specific contexts; like when you're meeting friends of friends at a party. Even then, you'll see the universal "arms slightly open" gesture that's basically asking, "hug okay?" before anyone moves in. When we do hug acquaintances, it's typically the safe side-hug, minimal body contact, quick squeeze, done.

Now, here's where things get interesting. Even in sexually open environments like lifestyle parties, where people literally gather to fuck around with friends, acquaintances, and strangers the same basic rules apply at first. Sure, friends might be more huggy right off the bat, but with people you've just met? You're still starting with handshakes and working your way up the touch ladder.

The key thing to understand is that context matters but consent always matters more. Whether you're at a church potluck or a sex party, you read the room and you ask; either verbally or through clear body language, before you touch someone.

Flirtatious touch is like everything flirty, it's playful and requires reading the situation. Safe places to briefly touch someone are forearms, shoulders, and knees. Women often respond positively to flirting by placing a hand on the other person's forearm or upper arm briefly. Classic example: "Oh, you're bad!" *laughs and lightly pushes his arm*; pushing him away while signaling she wants to keep talking.

Here's the reality: because we live in a gendered society, women initiating touch first is more socially acceptable than men doing it. This isn't a hard rule, but it's the cultural norm. The key thing for men to understand is that by the time most women reach adulthood, they've dealt with countless unwanted advances and genuinely scary situations because of how other men behaved. Many of those situations involved being touched without consent, so be careful. Really read the room before initiating touch, keep it light, and stick to non-sexual areas.

The escalation stages:

Stage one: Arms, shoulders, knees

Stage two: Previous areas plus hands, wrists, thighs above the knee, face/cheeks

Stage three: Neck, ears, inner thighs. At this point flirting becomes foreplay and can involve kissing and more intimate touches

Remember: mixed signals, unclear signals, and clear "no" signals mean back the fuck off. If alcohol &/or drugs are involved everyone's judgment gets impaired, so err on the side of caution and keep your hands to yourself, especially if you're a guy. Consent isn't just for sex; it starts with that first touch.

CHAPTER SIX

Porn

The Real Deal on Porn: It's Entertainment, Not Education

Look, porn isn't the devil, but it sure as hell isn't sex ed either. Here's what you need to know: porn is entertainment, period. It's designed to get you off, not teach you how to get someone else off. Treating it like a how-to guide is like learning to drive from watching Fast & Furious. It's entertaining as hell, but you'll crash and burn if you try that shit in real life.

Here's a few things you won't learn from porn:

The Magic Minute Myth: Porn makes it look like 30 seconds of halfhearted oral will have her climbing the walls. Spoiler alert: it won't. Most women need way more time to get warmed up, let alone reach the finish line. Take your time, pay attention, and for fuck's sake, don't treat it like a race.

The Screaming Orgasm Fantasy: Not everyone turns into a howler monkey when they cum. Some people grunt, some go silent, some moan like they're tasting the world's best pizza. You've got to read your partner, not follow some imaginary script or expect a performance worthy of an Oscar.

The Penetration Obsession: Here's a hard truth, most women don't come from fucking alone. Yeah, they might love it, but it's usually not what gets them across the finish line. Men, listen up: the clit is your best friend. There are a thousand ways to give it attention during sex, so get creative. Or check out some of the resources at the back for ideas.

The Missing Toys: Mainstream porn acts like toys don't exist, but in real life, they're MVP teammates. Don't be intimidated; they're tools, not competition.

Time Dilation: In porn the guy stays hard for literal hours, lasts hours and can control his orgasm for the ever entertaining money shot. However, most men cum between 3-7 minutes of direct fucking. Also, the male orgasm is not the end of the play date. There are plenty of other ways to continue playing, using your mouth and hands or toys can take the fun past one person's orgasm. So direct P in V sex doesn't last hours, the whole encounter can last hours but that involves foreplay, oral sex, anal play, cuddling, whatever else you can think of to make each other feel good. And there are breaks! Porn doesn't show taking a breather after an orgasm or two. Or going to the bathroom, having a water or a snack break, or quick nap before getting back to it.

Communication! In porn you rarely see the kind of communication needed to accurately express what makes you feel good; or what checking in with your partner/s looks like. The actors just seamlessly move from one position to the next. This is because it's all been mapped out ahead of time. Lube has been applied, douches have been douched, butts have been warmed up. You don't see breaks because they are edited out.

Here's the thing; most guys' first exposure to sex comes from porn or Hollywood's version of it. This quickly becomes their blueprint for how real sex should go, and that's where everything goes sideways.

Real sex is messy. It involves more communication than a UN summit, constant position adjustments, lube (your new best friend), weird sounds, farts, queefs, sweat and other bodily fluids, and about a thousand tiny course corrections to find your groove. If you can laugh at the awkward stuff, you're already winning. It sets a playful tone and helps everyone relax into the actual point of all this: pleasure. That doesn't mean there aren't moments of cinema worthy passion but expect those to be moments not the whole encounter.

As I've said before, people really fuck up by making orgasm the "goal." That's like trying to fall asleep by thinking really hard about sleeping. The pressure kills the fun for everyone. One person stresses about finishing, which makes finishing harder, then they spiral thinking their partner is getting bored or working too hard. Meanwhile, the other person feels like they're being graded on their performance, which gets them in their head about whether they're any good at this. It's a stress cycle that sucks the life out of what should be fun.

So, here's your takeaway: use porn like a sex toy, not a roadmap. Watch it alone to figure out what turns you on and enjoy some solo playtime. Watch it together to get turned on, maybe discover what fantasies you both have, or just enjoy the show. But don't expect your bedroom to look like a porn set. Porn stars are called adult actors/actresses for a reason. It's a performance, not a documentary.

The goal isn't to fuck like porn stars. It's to connect, have fun, figure out what turns you and your partner on, and enjoy the literal fuck out of each other. Make your own show.

Not all porn is created equal. There's porn for literally every kink, fantasy, and fetish under the sun. But here's the thing; most mainstream porn is basically the McDonald's of sex: cheap, fast, and designed for mass consumption, not quality. I've got no problem with McDonald's when I want fast food; but it would be ridiculous to try to sell a McDonald's cheeseburger as a gourmet meal.

Another hard truth of the matter is mainstream porn has a history of seriously mistreating women. Too much of it treats female performers like fuck dolls instead of human beings who deserve respect, fair pay, and agency over their own bodies. Yeah, you'll hear this criticism mostly from people who think all porn is evil because they believe sex for fun is sinful. I don't buy that bullshit conclusion, but they're not wrong about the industry's ugly history of exploitation and abuse.

But wait there's good news too! As more people stop being weird about sex, there's been a push toward more ethical production across the board. The leaders of this movement call it feminist porn; others just call it doing business right. Before you roll your eyes thinking it's all soft-focus lesbian scenes with lots of feelings, pump the brakes. Feminist porn isn't about who's fucking who. It's about who's calling the shots, how everyone gets treated while making the film as well as how everyone is portrayed in the scene.

We're talking fair wages, enthusiastic consent, realistic bodies, diverse performers, and sex that actually looks like people enjoying themselves instead of performing for some dude's alpha male fantasy. The performers have input on what they're comfortable doing, there's communication about boundaries, and everyone goes home feeling good about the work they did.

Think of it like the difference between a burger joint that pays living wages and sources quality ingredients versus one that cuts every corner. Both make burgers, but the experience is totally different. Same with porn. When everyone involved is treated with respect and the focus is on authentic pleasure, it shows. Admittedly, it can be more expensive; but it's better for the industry, the sex positive community, and your own mental health while enjoying porn.

Check the appendix for where to find the good stuff, your libido and your conscience will thank you.

CHAPTER SEVEN

Kink

Kink isn't just one thing. It's a lifestyle, a set of sexual practices, and an identity, sometimes all at once. At its core, kink refers to sexual and relationship practices that are outside the conventional playbook, encompassing everything from light bondage and role-playing to complex power exchange relationships and specific fetishes. It's a deviation from the standard narrative similar to the LGBTQ community. However, not all gay people are kinky, and not all kinky people are gay. It is another way people write their own story about sexuality and relationships.

Most people exploring kink first think of BDSM. Bondage, dominance, sadism, and masochism. But those are just the visible surface the rest of the world sees. Kink encompasses way more than that: restraint enthusiasts, impact play (spanking, flogging), sensory play (temperature, textures), age play, pet play, latex fetishes, foot worship, and countless other expressions. While some people are drawn to physical sensations, others explore the psychological aspects of power exchange and safely explore being "abused." Many also enjoy the ritual and ceremony that can surround kink activities.

In kink, consent is so much more than a word, it's a moral principal. Often people think kink is about ignoring boundaries or about a person letting someone do whatever they want to them. It's actually the total opposite. Kinky people treat consent not just as a legal requirement, but as a personal moral principle that guides everything they do.

Everyone involved must understand exactly what's happening, agree to it beforehand, discuss their limits and boundaries, and retain the power to stop everything immediately. This isn't just about the big stuff. It covers everything from what names someone is comfortable being called, to which words are ok to use, to which body parts are off limits, to specific types of touch they do or don't want (like tickling, which can be surprisingly intense for some people), to how much degradation they can handle.

The kink community has incredibly high standards around consent because they have to. When your activities involve things like restraints, impact tools, psychological power exchange, or putting someone in vulnerable positions, there's no room for ambiguity. While boundary violations in any context can cause serious harm and trauma, the margin for error becomes particularly narrow when deliberately manipulating power dynamics for pleasure. This requires incredible communication and trust to be fulfilling for all.

People's reputations in kink communities are directly tied to how well they respect consent, and these communities talk. When someone violates boundaries, word gets around fast, and that person will find themselves shunned at events, in online groups, and social circles. This isn't just social drama; it's community self-defense.

Because kink is already misunderstood and stigmatized by broader society, anything that makes it seem unsafe or abusive threatens everyone in the community. One person's bad behavior can fuel a moral panic that affects everyone's ability to practice safely and openly. This requires additional vigilance because predators and abusive people sometimes use the guise of being "kinky" as cover for genuinely harmful behavior; like claiming that abuse is just their "kink" or that victims consented to activities they clearly didn't agree to. So, the community polices itself aggressively. Consent violators don't just lose partners, they are purged.

Every experience or "scene" starts with negotiation, and this isn't a quick "you cool with this?" conversation. It's a detailed discussion about what everyone wants to happen, what emotional experience they are looking for, what they absolutely don't want, what their hard limits are versus their soft limits, what they're curious about trying, and what aftercare they'll need. Someone might want to feel powerful, vulnerable, cared for, or challenged and that emotional component is just as important as the physical activities.

Hard limits are non-negotiable boundaries; things that are completely off the table. Soft limits are things someone isn't sure about or doesn't want right now but might be open to exploring later or under different circumstances. Good kink partners respect both equally.

Intense kink scenes often involve emotional and physical vulnerability that requires transition time afterward. Aftercare includes debriefing. Honest conversation about what felt good, what didn't work, and what might be adjusted next time. At a party where participants are strangers, this may be a short brief. In a relationship with a developed dynamic, it might last much longer and include physical comfort like blankets, water, gentle touch, emotional reassurance, or just quiet time to process what happened. It's acknowledgment that intense experiences, even positive ones, affect people and they need support coming back to baseline.

It's kinda funny that communities that are often seen as "deviant" or "unsafe" actually have more explicit, thoughtful approaches to consent and communication than mainstream dating culture. While vanilla couples often stumble through sexual miscommunications and unspoken assumptions, kink communities have developed sophisticated frameworks for discussing desires, boundaries, and ongoing consent.

In a world where regular communication is already ambiguous as fuck, this kind of detailed, ongoing dialogue would benefit most vanilla relationships as well. It's worth thinking about what the rest of us could learn from that.

Safe Words and Power Exchange

The key insight kinky people understand is that consent can be revoked at any time, even in the middle of intense scenes. That's where safe words come in; agreed upon words or signals that communicate real needs separate from the role-play. The most common system is "yellow" meaning slow down, check in; and "red", stop and change activities; and then whatever word you come up with, for example "pineapple" means stop everything now. Some people also use nonverbal signals like dropping an object or specific hand gestures for situations where they can't speak.

In power exchange dynamics, someone might be role-playing resistance or saying "no" as part of the fantasy, so safe words let them communicate their real feelings versus their character's feelings. When someone uses a safe word, the roleplay stops immediately and check in happens; no questions, no negotiation, no pushing through "just a little more." This creates an incredible level of trust that actually allows people to explore more intense experiences than they'd ever feel safe doing otherwise.

The counterintuitive magic of safe words is that having a guaranteed "escape hatch" lets people go deeper into vulnerable territory. When you know you can stop anything instantly and be heard, you can surrender control more completely or push your own boundaries more boldly. It's the safety net that makes the high wire act possible.

Safe words aren't just for intense kink scenes either. Many couples use them for all kinds of situations. During play with other couples, when a social interaction isn't working and they need to extract themselves gracefully, or when they need to pause and reconnect during partner swapping. Any time you want crystal clear communication about when something needs to change, safe words cut through ambiguity and give everyone an easy out. You can even use safe words when we need to take a breather during an argument and return later.

Top/Bottom vs. Dom/Sub: Not the Same Thing

Top/bottom refers to physical position and action, not power dynamics. The top is the one doing something to someone else like, penetrating, spanking, tying up, etc. This applies to all kinds of activities, not just anal sex. The bottom is the one receiving; being penetrated, spanked, or tied up. It's purely about who is giving and who is receiving the physical activity.

Often the top is also the dom and the bottom is also the sub, which aligns with what people instinctively expect. But top/bottom is completely separate from dom/sub dynamics. One is about physical positioning, the other is about psychological power and control. A dominant person might be physically on the bottom, directing and controlling a submissive partner who's doing the physical work on top. This is called "topping from the bottom." The bottom is receiving the physical activity but maintaining psychological control over what happens. I know, the terms don't match up. Logically it should be "doming from the bottom." There are other books on the weirdness of language; for our purposes, don't over think it.

Some concrete examples: In male/male interactions, the top might be the one penetrating or having their penis sucked, while the bottom is being penetrated or doing the sucking. In lesbian interactions, the top might be the one using a strap-on, doing the fingering, or performing oral sex, while the bottom receives these activities. For trans folks, these roles can be defined by the specific acts involved rather than assumptions based on anatomy. A trans woman might top by penetrating with her penis, or bottom by receiving anal or oral sex, regardless of how others might categorize her body or whose "in charge."

In all these scenarios, the person in the physically receptive role could easily be the dominant partner. They tell their partner exactly how to fuck them, instructing more or less intensity, and directing the entire encounter. The physical position doesn't determine who has the power. You can have dominant bottoms, submissive tops, as well as dominant tops and submissive bottoms, and everything in between. Understanding this distinction helps clarify what people actually want. Someone might be interested in bottoming physically but want to maintain control or want to top physically while being told exactly what to do.

Dom/sub refers to psychological power and control, not physical position. The dominant partner (dom) takes charge of the scene, makes decisions about what happens, and controls the pace and intensity. The submissive partner (sub) yields control, follows direction, and finds pleasure in being guided or commanded. It's about who has the psychological authority in the dynamic. This topping from the bottom shows how psychological control can flow independently of physical position.

"Switch" refers to being able to dom and sub depending on your partner or mood. "Verse" means you can top or bottom, again, depending on the situation. Don't confuse these: dom/sub is about who's got the psychological power, while top/bottom is about who's doing what physically.

This shit matters when you're talking to potential partners. If I say I'm verse, I'm telling you I'm down to give or receive. You might lean more toward one side; that's totally normal. Someone could say "I'm verse but honestly, the whole dom/sub thing doesn't do it for me" and that's perfectly valid. The same goes for saying, "I'm a bottom" or "I'm a top."

Here's the thing: you can have amazing sex as verse partners without any power games at all. Both people communicate what they want, meet each other's needs, and nobody has to be "in charge." Bottom line: bottoms are receiving, tops are giving, and verse folks do whatever the fuck feels right.

Sexuality is a spectrum, not a checklist. You don't have to fit perfectly into any box, but if a label helps you communicate what you want, use it. The whole point is figuring out what works for you and your partner, not following some rulebook.

Impact Play: The Roller Coaster of Kink

Impact play is exactly what it sounds like - hitting someone for fun, theirs and yours. Spanking, flogging, cropping, or anything else that makes contact with skin in delicious ways. Now, before you roll your eyes, here's the science: pain and pleasure live right next to each other in your brain, just like anxiety and excitement. That's why roller coasters are thrilling instead of just terrifying, and why a good spanking can make you wet instead of just sore.

Here's the crucial difference: when you got spanked as a kid, that was punishment designed to teach you a lesson. Impact play? That's about sensation, connection, and getting off. No lesson required, just consensual adults making each other feel amazing (even when it hurts).

Impact play doesn't have to be painful; it's about sensation, and it's a spectrum. You can use:

Soft sensations: Feathers, silk, gentle fingertips, or light tapping

Thuddy impacts: Paddles, floggers with wide tails, or open palms that create deep, spreading sensation

Stingy impacts: Crops, canes, or single-tail whips that create sharp, focused pain

Temperature play: Ice, wax, warming oils, or implements that have been heated or cooled

Texture variations: Studded paddles, textured gloves, or rough rope

The magic is in building intensity. You start soft and work your way up. Always. This isn't just about being nice; it's about physiology. Your body needs time to produce endorphins and get into that headspace where pain becomes pleasure.

Tools of the Trade :   Different tools create different sensations:

Hands: The classic. Immediate feedback, perfect control, and intimate connection. Plus, they're always available.

Paddles: Create broad, thuddy impacts. Great for beginners because they're hard to fuck up.

Floggers: Multiple tails that can be used gently for warm-up or intensely for serious impact. The sensation depends on the material, leather thuds, rubber stings.

Crops: Precise, stingy impacts. Excellent control but require more skill.

Canes: Advanced territory. Intense, precise, and absolutely requires proper technique.

Single-tails: Expert level only. These can cause serious damage in inexperienced hands.

Safety and Technique

This is where people fuck up royally. Impact play looks easy, just hit someone, right? Wrong. There's anatomy to learn (stay away from kidneys, spine, and joints), techniques to master (how to swing without torquing your wrist), and skills to develop (reading your partner's body language, building intensity properly).

You've got to learn anatomy. Know where it's safe to hit and where it absolutely isn't. Start every session with warm-up impacts, even if you've played before. Have clear safe words. Remember, "yellow" for slow down, "red" for stop immediately. Check in regularly, especially with new partners. Aftercare is mandatory, endorphins crash hard after intense scenes

Impact play pairs beautifully with power dynamics. The physical sensation combined with the psychological elements of control and submission can be incredibly intense. The dominant gets to orchestrate their partner's experience, while the submissive gets to surrender and receive. It's intimate as hell when done right.

Please, for the love of all that's kinky, don't show up at a party with a bag full of floggers claiming you're an expert when you've only practiced on pillows. Everyone can tell, it makes the whole community look bad, and more importantly, you could seriously hurt someone. Don't be that asshole. Take classes. Practice. Learn from experienced players. Your future partners (and their marked up skin) will thank you.

Power Play Dynamics

Power play is the branch of kink that gets into dominance and submission without necessarily requiring pain like you'd see in impact play. It's all about exploring and flipping traditional power structures in consensual, hot-as-fuck ways. Some classic dynamics include:

Master/Slave: The most intense power exchange, often involving complete authority transfer within negotiated boundaries

Daddy/Baby: Caretaking with authority (and yeah, it's not always about age - more about nurturing control)

Brat/Brat Tamer: For when you want to be a little shit and get put in your place through discipline and structure

Big/Little: Age play that explores different headspaces and care dynamics, from playful to deeply regressive

Owner/Pet: Animal roleplay with training, rewards, and behavioral expectations

Boss/Employee: Professional power dynamics taken into intimate territory

Teacher/Student: Academic authority with lessons, rules, consequences, and rewards

Mommy/Boy or Girl: Maternal dominance focusing on care, guidance, and sometimes humiliation

Hunter/Prey: Predator/victim dynamics involving chase, capture, and control.

Goddess/Worshipper: Divine authority where the dominant is literally worshipped and served

Captor/Captive: Consensual non-consent scenarios with imprisonment themes

Alpha/Beta or Omega: Borrowing from omegaverse fiction, exploring biological hierarchy composed of dominant alphas, neutral betas, and submissive omegas, dictates social interactions, particularly in romantic and sexual contexts

Here's the thing about power dynamics, they're not just bedroom roleplay. They tap into some deep psychological shit about control, surrender, trust, and transformation. Some people get off on giving up control because it's the only time they can truly let go. Others need to be in charge because that's where they feel most authentic and caring.

The beauty is in the flip, maybe you're a CEO who needs to be told what to do for once, or a people-pleaser who discovers they love making someone else submit. Power play lets you explore parts of yourself that regular life doesn't always accommodate.

There are tons more variations because humans are creative as hell when it comes to power and sex, and really, most people end up creating their own hybrid dynamics that work for their specific relationship.

Collaring: The Kinky Wedding Ring

Collaring is serious business. Think of it as the kink world's version of marriage. It's usually a formal ceremony where a dominant gives their submissive a collar, symbolizing consensual ownership. Now, before anyone gets their panties in a twist, we're talking about the same kind of "ownership" you have with a beloved pet. You care for them, protect them, and guide them because you love them.

When someone accepts a collar, they're agreeing to let their dominant control certain aspects of their life. Maybe it's what they wear to events, who they play with at parties, or how they handle household tasks. The specifics depend on what they've negotiated.

Here's the crucial part that too many people fuck up: the dominant isn't just getting a sexy plaything. They're taking on massive responsibility. They're committing to their sub's physical, emotional, and sexual wellbeing. They need to nourish, train, guide, and protect. Just like you would with any pet under your care.

Keep in mind, even collared subs can withdraw consent. If your "owner" is treating you like shit, putting you in danger, or ignoring your needs, that collar comes off. No exceptions. Good dominants understand this; and shitty ones don't deserve subs.

Most people only get collared by one person at a time, even if they play with others. The collar represents primary ownership, and it's typically the dominant's job to vet and approve (or even orchestrate) their sub's other encounters.

Protocol: How Deep Does the Rabbit Hole Go?

Protocol is basically how much of your regular life gets wrapped up in the power exchange. It's the difference between bedroom-only kink and living it 24/7, or somewhere in between.

Low Protocol: Power exchange happens during scenes and play time. The rest of the time, you're equals handling adult responsibilities like jobs, bills, and whose turn it is to take out the trash.

High Protocol: The power dynamic extends into daily life. We're talking rules about posture, speech, when you can sit, what you can eat, the works. Sounds intense? It fucking is. Also, it's not realistic for most people because adult life requires independence and decision-making that high protocol can complicate to unrealistic levels.

Scene Protocol: This is where most people play. During a scene, high protocol might mean sitting perfectly still in a corner until given permission to move or following elaborate rules about eye contact and speech. Break a rule? There are sexy consequences. But when the scene is over, including aftercare, the power exchange is over. You are equals again.

Remember: no matter what protocol level you're playing at, consent doesn't disappear. Dominants are still responsible for their subs' wellbeing; physical, mental, emotional, and sexual. That responsibility doesn't get lighter just because someone's wearing a collar; in fact, it gets heavier.

Beyond the Fuzzy Handcuffs

Ah, the ole' fuzzy handcuffs from Spencer's. Cute, but that's just kindergarten-level restraint play. The real world of bondage ranges from intricate rope work to being chained to a St. Andrew's Cross, or even just having your wrists tied with a necktie above your head (hello, 50 Shades). There's a whole spectrum of ways to give up or take control.

Don't Fuck Around with Safety. This isn't negotiable. When someone can't move freely, safe words aren't just nice to have; they're lifelines, and they must be honored immediately. No exceptions, no "just a little longer," no "you can take a little more," no bullshit. Period.

Here's what you need to know: some knots tighten when you move or struggle (which is kind of the point) and holding certain positions too long can actually damage nerves and circulation. The person doing the tying, known as "the rigger," is responsible for their partner's safety at all times. The person getting tied up, known as "the rope bunny," or just "bunny" is responsible for speaking up when something's wrong.

Keep safety shears nearby. These are blunt-tipped hospital scissors that cut through anything. If shit goes sideways, you need to get someone free fast, not fumble with knots for ten minutes.

Pro tip: Remember, safe words don't have to only be used for full stop. "Yellow" can mean "getting close to my limit," "red" means "no harder than that but don't stop," and "pineapple" means full stop and check in. Figure out your words beforehand and stick to it.

Vulnerability is the real kink. Here's the thing people don't talk about enough. Giving up control over your body is incredibly vulnerable and can be genuinely therapeutic. But because being helpless can so easily flip from hot to traumatic, this is not the time for stupid jokes about leaving someone tied up or pretending to rob them or whatever other intrusive thought pops into your head. Breaking that trust when someone's literally tied up can fuck them up way worse than most other bedroom mistakes. Don't be that asshole.

So What's Shibari All About?

Let's talk about shibari (pronounced she-BAH-ree). It literally means "to tie" in Japanese, and it's had quite the journey. What started as a way for samurai to restrain prisoners (called Hojōjutsu back then) has transformed into something completely different: a consensual, creative way for partners to connect that's equal parts art form and intimate experience. Think of it as painting, but your canvas is your partner's body and your brush is rope. Pretty cool, right?

Shibari isn't just about tying someone up and calling it a day. There's a whole visual feast happening that celebrates beautiful imperfection (the Japanese call this *wabi-sabi*) and plays with the contrast between rope and skin. Ever notice how a shadow can be as striking as the object casting it? That's the Japanese concept of *ma* – the powerful space between things. When you see rope against skin creating patterns and shadows, you'll get what I mean.

For rope, most folks go with natural fibers like jute or hemp – about as thick as your pinky and long enough to get creative with. These have the right grip so knots stay put, plus they feel amazing against skin. Not into natural fibers? Cotton, linen, or synthetic ropes work just fine and each brings its own feel to the party.

Some terms:

- **Kinbaku** (say it: keen-BAH-koo): Sometimes used interchangeably with shibari, though some rope nerds (and I mean that lovingly!) will tell you it focuses more on the emotional connection
- **Single and double column ties**: Your bread-and-butter moves for tying wrists, ankles, or thighs
- **Friction-based knots**: These are your friends! They stay put without tightening up and causing a panic
- **Harnesses**: Those gorgeous webs of rope that wrap around the chest or torso
- **Suspension**: The advanced stuff where you're actually lifting someone off the ground. Definitely not where you start!

Imagine having pressure points activated all over your body while feeling both hugged tight and completely exposed at the same time. That's the sensory rollercoaster of shibari. You've got rope sliding across skin, growing tension as each tie comes together, and that unique feeling of "I could struggle, but why would I want to?" Many people drift into "rope space," or "subspace;" kind of like a runner's high but without the running.

The mental side is just as intense. Shibari keeps you totally present. There's no thinking about your inbox when rope's involved. It's a trust fall on steroids, perfect for getting back in your body when you've spent too much time in your head, and lets you express things that words can't touch. Sometimes the rope says what conversation can't.

Here's the players, you've got the rigger (or *nawashi* if you're fancy) doing the tying, and the model (also called bunny or bottom) getting tied. But here's the thing, it's not a one-way street where one person does everything. It's more like dancing, with constant communication and working together. Perfect knots mean nothing if you're not connecting with your partner.

Keep it safe and consensual. Wrapping someone in rope comes with serious responsibility. Blood flow matters: "Can you wiggle those fingers?" isn't small talk. Numb limbs or weird skin colors mean blood isn't flowing right. Some nerves run close to the surface at wrists, armpits, and the back of knees. Squish these wrong and you're looking at damage that lasts way longer than your session.

Body positioning that feels fine for five minutes might be torture after twenty. Always keep safety scissors within reach and know how to get someone out fast. This isn't the time to fumble with knots.

The pre-session chat matters: what you're into, what's off-limits, any physical issues. "How are you doing?" should be your most common phrase during rope time. Aftercare is not optional! Cuddling, hydration, processing the experience, whatever helps you both transition back to regular life.

Nobody becomes a shibari master overnight. Find actual people who know their shit to learn from, YouTube only takes you so far. Practice basic ties and learn where nerves and blood vessels are (way sexier than it sounds when someone's tied up in your ropes). Get good at talking while tying; and join workshops where you can learn from the community.

Shibari comes from Japan, and that cultural context matters. Remember where these practices come from, know the difference between appreciating a culture and appropriating it, take time to learn the history, and support Japanese educators when possible. Don't be that person who slaps on a kimono and calls themselves "Rope Master."

Shibari can spice things up by creating new sensations when movement is restricted, making foreplay last longer (there's rushing intricate rope work), adding serious visual appeal, and playing with power dynamics in a structured way. Whether you use it as part of sex or keep it separate as its own experience, it offers this amazing combo of artistic expression, sensory exploration, and deep connection that many people find absolutely mind-blowing. It's like finding a whole new way to communicate with partners. Just with knots instead of words.

Consensual Non-Consent (CNC): The Ultimate Mind Fuck

CNC stands for Consensual Non-Consent, and it's exactly as complicated as it sounds. This is roleplay that explores having your power stripped away. The fantasy of being "forced" while actually being in complete control. It's psychological BDSM at its most intense, and it's not for beginners or people who half-ass their communication.

Let's Be Crystal Fucking Clear. If you're interested in CNC, that does NOT mean you want to be sexually assaulted. Read that again. The fantasy of controlled powerlessness is completely different from actual violation. CNC is about exploring surrender and fear in a safe container with someone you trust absolutely.

Even if you're actively involved in CNC scenes, that doesn't give anyone, including your regular CNC partner, permission to take advantage of you without explicit consent for that specific encounter. Consent doesn't transfer between situations or people.

Here's the mind-bending part: in CNC, the "victim" actually holds all the real power. It's a controlled loss of control. They're the one who decides when, where, how, and with whom this happens. Even if they choose to let their partner decide some of those aspects, they retain complete control through safe words, safe signals, and the fundamental right to stop everything immediately.

Think of it like the roller coaster analogy again; you're strapped in and plummeting toward what feels like certain death, but you know the engineers designed it to be safe. The thrill comes from that temporary suspension of control while actually being completely protected.

CNC requires planning! You need to discuss:

Boundaries and limits: What acts are okay? What's absolutely off-limits? What might be okay later but not now?

The scenario: Home invasion? Sleeping partner? Reluctant partner? The basic "plot" needs to be agreed upon.

Safe words and signals: Standard red/yellow, plus physical signals for when mouths are occupied. Some people use objects to drop or specific hand or body movements.

Aftercare planning: CNC can be emotionally intense. Plan for immediate aftercare and check-ins over the following days.

Duration and escape routes: How long might this last? How does it end? What if real life intervenes?

Here's some common CNC scenarios

Sleep play: Partner initiates sex while you're sleeping. Sounds simple, but requires detailed discussion about timing, acts, and wake-up protocols.

Home invasion: Elaborate roleplay involving "breaking in" and "taking" someone. Requires serious planning about safe words, neighbors, and realistic vs. fantasy elements.

Reluctant partner: Roleplaying initial resistance that "breaks down." Heavy on the psychological elements and requires excellent communication skills.

Blackmail/coercion: Power-based scenarios involving threats or consequences. Advanced territory that requires serious trust.

CNC can serve different psychological needs:

Surrender: For people who carry a lot of responsibility, the fantasy of having all choice removed can be liberating.

Reclaiming power: Some assault survivors find that controlling their own "violation" helps them process trauma. This should ideally be done with therapeutic support, obviously with the therapist helping with planning and debriefing afterward. No therapist should be volunteering for the "predator" role!

Taboo exploration: Safely exploring fantasies that would be horrific in reality.

Intensity seeking: The emotional and physical intensity of CNC can be addictive for sensation seekers.

Red Flags and Reality Checks
Don't do CNC if:

- You're new to BDSM or don't have excellent communication skills
- You're with a partner you don't trust completely
- Either partner has untreated trauma that might be triggered
- You're using it to avoid dealing with actual assault or abuse
- You can't clearly articulate your boundaries and limits

Warning signs of bad CNC:

- Partner pressures you into it
- No discussion of limits or safe words
- Partner gets angry when you use safe words
- No aftercare or emotional support
- Partner uses CNC as an excuse for actual assault

CNC is psychological kink for advanced players who have their shit together. It requires absolute trust, meticulous planning, and excellent communication. When done right, it can be incredibly intense and fulfilling. When done wrong, it becomes actual assault.

If you're curious about CNC, start small. Maybe begin with some light restraint and "reluctance" roleplay before moving to more elaborate scenarios. Take classes, read books, and for fuck's sake, choose your partners carefully. This isn't casual hookup territory. This is intimate, vulnerable stuff that requires people who genuinely care about your wellbeing.

The Darker Side: When Kink Gets Extreme

Look, we need to talk about the stuff that makes even experienced kinksters pause. This is the hardcore territory: scat play, blood play, water sports, extreme degradation, psychological torture, snuff fantasies, and physical torture. These aren't your typical "spank me harder" kinks. They're intense, potentially dangerous, and definitely not for everyone.

Here's my honest take: I'm not into this. It's a genuine turn-off for me, and I don't have the personal experience to guide you safely through these practices. But here's the thing, just because something isn't my cup of tea doesn't mean it's wrong or that the people who are into it are fucked up. I'm just not your guide here. I could bullshit my way through explaining edge play I've never done, but that would be dangerous and irresponsible. These kinks often involve serious health risks, complex psychological dynamics, and safety protocols that I haven't lived through. You deserve better than someone half-assing their way through advice that could literally harm you.

What I Will Say

If you're drawn to extreme kink:

- You're not broken or sick
- Find mentors who actually practice what you're interested in
- Take safety more seriously than you've ever taken anything in your life
- Start slow and work with experienced partners
- Have medical knowledge or access to people who do

Red flags in extreme kink communities:

- Anyone who dismisses safety protocols as "vanilla concerns"
- Partners who push you toward more extreme practices than you're ready for
- Groups that shame you for having limits or using safe words
- People who confuse fantasy with reality

Finding Better Resources

Look for:

- **Specialized communities** for your specific interests (FetLife groups, local munches)

- **Educational resources** written by people who actually practice these kinks
- **Medical professionals** who understand kink (yes, they exist)
- **Experienced practitioners** willing to mentor safely

Don't learn extreme edge play from porn, random internet articles, YouTube, or people who've only fantasized about it. The stakes are too high for amateur hour.

I'm not going to pretend to be an expert on shit I don't do. That's not kink shaming, that's being honest about my limitations so you can find people who can actually help you explore safely. Everyone deserves accurate information and safe practices, especially when the kinks get dangerous.

Your interests are valid. Just make sure you're getting guidance from people who know what the fuck they're talking about.

CHAPTER EIGHT

Ethical Non-Monogamy

Ethical Non-Monogamy: More Than One Way to Love

Ethical Non-Monogamy (ENM) is an umbrella term that covers any relationship structure outside the "one person forever" model that has become the standard narrative in most, but not all, cultures. It's not about being unable to commit or wanting to fuck around without consequences. It's about consciously choosing relationship structures that actually meet the needs and desires of all the people involved. And boy are there many options to choose from!

There is a fairy tale we've all been brought up on: that there is one perfect person out there who will be your lover, best friend, therapist, adventure buddy, co-parent, financial partner, and emotional support system all rolled into one. They'll share your sexual interests, political views, life goals, and sense of humor. Oh, and you'll both want exactly the same level of social interaction, alone time, and Netflix preferences.

Totally realistic, right? Now, this kind of one person forever connection does happen and some people are very happy that way. It's just not *the only way*; and may not actually be the majority way either.... Seriously, if it's not *the only way* to be happy, why are we trying to fit our needs into someone else's box?

Here's what couple's therapists spend most of their time dealing with: mismatched sex drives, different money philosophies, conflicting political views, incompatible social needs, and disagreements about everything from career priorities to how to load the dishwasher.

When combined with all the other life stresses out there, it's easy to see how a person can slowly slide into a "what they don't know won't hurt them" mindset. Be it sneaking a bit of cake at night, or glossing over that flirty conversation with your coworker, or hitting up some porn while the spouse is shopping, to full on cheating and affairs. The truth is *it is* easier to just get your needs met on your own rather than talking it through with a partner that doesn't share that desire. It's not sustainable, but it is easier in the moment.

All those conflicts couple's therapists untangle aren't character flaws. These are conflicts that monogamous and non-monogamous people will struggle with regardless. The idea that "good" relationships will not have any struggles is unhelpful at best. The idea of struggling well, now, that is what real life is made of. Partnerships are more about *collaborating with*, rather than *compromising for*.

The fairy tale that we've been sold with the "and they lived happily ever after" narrative we've grown up on is that none of these conflicts will arise in your relationship if it's with *"the one."* That after the dramatic crisis of defining the relationship and committing to our partner, the drama of our story is over. Except in real life, it's not. Bills still need to be paid next month. New people will come into your life. Job changes, births, deaths, accidents and illnesses will all happen. And what got you guys through that first define the relationship crisis will likely not get you through all of life's inevitable crises. What will get you through? Honesty and communication, with yourself and with others.

Why Monogamy Isn't Magic

Let's take attraction as an example. Most romantic comedies treat attraction to multiple people as a crisis that needs resolving. You must choose and choose well! But what if the crisis isn't having feelings, but the *assumption* that having feelings is automatically a problem?

However much in love a couple is when they first meet, there will at some point in the future be an attraction to someone else. Maybe not an acted on attraction, maybe just a good looking celebrity on TV. More likely, a new colleague at work, your kid's new teacher this year, a friend of a friend that you met at happy hour, or something else equally exciting. You will feel yourself "drawn to them" and conflicted because you've already had the "I found my person" experience. Here's the thing, there are attractive people in the world. You will cross paths with them. Expecting yourself to not feel attraction after a commitment is like expecting the tiger's stripes to change to spots after mating. Finding yourself attracted to another person is **NORMAL**. Surprisingly, you can apply this reframe to so many other "crises." Feeling jealous, feeling angry, scared, bored, attractive, horny, sad, restless, excited, keep going. Feelings are normal. (Feelings will also lie to you, but that's a different section.) How you manage those feelings is where the monogamous narrative fucks people up.

The monogamous narrative says that if you have any unexpected or unacceptable feelings in your relationship *something is wrong*, and that the solution is to convince your partner to do something different to solve it. The monogamous narrative says that your partner is responsible for your feelings. If you are feeling attracted to someone else, it's your partner's responsibility to recapture your attention. If you're feeling bored, it's your partner's responsibility to excite you. If you're feeling horny it's your partner's responsibility to satiate you. This is the problem. As much as we would like to take responsibility for someone else's feelings we just can't. It's something that is out of our control. We can influence a person's feelings, but we can't control them. So, our response to our partner's feelings is better thought of as a collaboration rather than an obligation to change. I think of it like, I'm not responsible for my partner's feelings; but because I love her, I do care how she feels and will try to help. It can also be rephrased as, my partner is not responsible for my feelings but I do expect them to give a shit and try to help.

Sometimes that "help" looks like accepting that your partner finds other people attractive and asking them to reassure you that you are not less important to them because of it.

There Is Nothing Wrong with Monogamy

I'm not here to shit on monogamy. For many people, it's exactly what they want, the deep intimacy, shared life building, and exclusive connection that comes with focusing on one person. That's beautiful when it works.

But let's stop pretending it's the *only* valid relationship structure or that people who want something different are damaged, selfish, or commitment-phobic. Different people have different relationship needs, and there's no one-size-fits-all approach to love and connection.

You Should Read This Even If You're Monogamous.

Even if you have zero interest in multiple partners, the concepts in ENM can transform your relationship. Learning to communicate clearly about needs, negotiate boundaries, handle jealousy maturely, and build relationships intentionally rather than just defaulting to cultural scripts. That shit is relationship gold, regardless of how many people are involved. So, stick around, even if ENM isn't your thing. You might learn something that makes your one relationship even stronger.

Communication is a superpower. Here's the thing that might surprise you: people in successful ENM relationships often have better communication skills than a lot of monogamous couples. Why? Because you literally cannot navigate multiple relationships without being crystal clear about your needs, boundaries, and feelings.

ENM forces you to: Articulate what you actually want from relationships. Negotiate time, energy, and emotional resources. Deal with jealousy and insecurity head-on. Be honest about your limitations and capacity. Practice compersion (being happy about your partner's other relationships, sexual or otherwise.)

Plot twist: These skills would revolutionize most monogamous relationships too.

Understanding Polyamory: More Than Just Multiple Partners

Polyamory is the practice of having multiple romantic relationships with the full knowledge and consent of everyone involved. But here's what sets it apart from other forms of ethical non-monogamy (ENM): it's built on emotional connection and long-term commitment, not just sexual variety.

While swinging might be about having sex with other couples and open relationships might allow for casual hookups, polyamory is about developing full relationships with multiple people. We're talking about having another boyfriend or girlfriend who you actually date; going to movies, taking walks, meeting their family, dealing with their weird dishwasher-loading habits.

Polyamorous relationships include sex, sure, but that's just one component. You're building emotional connections, sharing life experiences, and yes, dealing with all the mundane relationship stuff that comes with actually caring about someone long-term.

This can be fucking amazing. Imagine having one partner who shares your financial values and family goals, but you disagree on everything from Netflix choices to gym importance. Then you have another partner who loves the same obscure horror films you do and will actually go hiking without complaining. Sexually, maybe your primary partner loves slow, connected bonding sex, while your other partner is into more adventurous fucking with different positions and power dynamics. It's not that one is "better," it's that the variety enriches your life in ways monogamy can't.

Thing is, this is next level shit. Having one partner is hard work. Now multiple that by however many partners you have. You're managing multiple birthdays, Valentine's Days, and holiday schedules. You're attending your metamour's (your partner's other partner) mom's retirement party. You're keeping track of multiple people's emotional needs, schedules, and relationship dynamics. And we haven't even gotten to jealousy yet!

Sometimes it's easier to watch your partner fucking someone else than it is to watch them build an emotional connection with another person. It hits different when you're used to being someone's only emotional anchor.

Types of Polyamory: Choose Your Own Adventure
Hierarchical Polyamory

There's a clear "primary" partnership (often married couples) and "secondary" relationships. Everyone knows where they stand. The primary relationship gets priority in major decisions, but that doesn't mean secondary relationships are just afterthoughts. However, let's be honest, people do sometimes leave primary partnerships for secondary ones, despite the supposed hierarchy. And of course, it's important to make sure the secondary partner's still feel cared for and valuable. There are many situations where a person has to disappoint one of their partners and which one will it be today and how will we decide…?

Relationship Anarchy

This style says, "fuck the hierarchy." Every relationship exists on its own terms without predetermined labels or rankings. You might spend Tuesday night with one partner and Friday with another, based on what feels right, not some arbitrary relationship ranking system.

This works especially well for "solo poly" people who maintain much of their day to day independence, such as living alone, having their own finances, their own support systems, while having multiple meaningful relationships. Not trying to build a traditional couple structure with anyone allows for much more freedom in how you obligate yourself in your relationships.

Kitchen Table Polyamory

Everyone gets to know everyone. When you become someone's partner, you're welcomed to the metaphorical "kitchen table" where all of that person's partners can meet, build their own friendships, and support each other's relationships.

For example, a husband and wife couple that have regular dinners with both their other partners at the same table, talk about schedules, dates and planning special events like birthdays together. It's a hippy utopia! And if there are kids in the family it's extremely helpful to have more responsible and loving adults in your village.

It sounds idealistic, but when it works, it creates a chosen family dynamic that can be incredibly supportive. When it doesn't work... well, that's a lot of awkward dinner parties.

Polyamory isn't for everyone, and it's definitely not a solution to existing relationship problems. It requires exceptional communication skills, time management abilities, and emotional intelligence. But for people who thrive on deep connections with multiple people and have the bandwidth to manage complex relationship networks, it can be deeply fulfilling.

Just know what you're signing up for before you dive in.

Open Relationships: Friends Who Fuck

The key difference between poly and open relationships is that open relationships are built around sexual connection rather than emotional entanglement. While polyamory is about developing full romantic relationships with multiple people, open relationships are about maintaining a primary partnership while having sexual connections outside of it.

Think of it this way: in polyamory, you might be planning weekend trips and meeting each other's parents. In open relationships, you're planning when to fuck and maybe grabbing dinner first.

The connections you have outside your primary relationship are predominantly sexual. Sure, there might be some light dating involved; drinks, dinner, getting to know each other, but everyone understands the end goal is sexual. You're not building toward moving in together or blending families.

These are friends with benefits or regular fuck buddies. You care about each other as people. You'll listen when they need to vent about work, you'll reschedule if they have a family emergency, you give a shit if they're having a rough day. But you're not deeply involved in each other's lives. You don't know their kids, you're not invited to family holidays, and you both understand that Mother's Day or Father's Day doesn't involve you. The friendship exists because you enjoy fucking each other and you do it somewhat regularly. Your day-to-day lives don't intersect much beyond that sexual connection.

Open relationships often involve staying active on dating apps and sites. People come and go naturally. You meet someone new, experience that rush of new relationship energy (NRE), go on dates, hook up regularly for weeks or months, and then life happens. Someone moves, gets busy with work, or just naturally drifts away.

No big breakup drama, no custody arrangements for shared friend groups. You find new fuck buddies, rinse and repeat. It's a cycle that works for people who enjoy variety, meeting new people, and the excitement of fresh sexual connections without the complexity of multiple romantic relationships. This setup also works well for people who want sexual variety and adventure while maintaining one primary emotional relationship. You get the thrill of new connections and different sexual experiences and have a secure emotional base in your primary partner.

It's also typically less time-intensive than polyamory. A fuck buddy relationship might be a few hours every couple of weeks, not the ongoing emotional labor of multiple full-time relationships.

Swinging: Couples Playing Together

What makes swinging special is that swinging is a specific type of open relationship focused on couples exchanging partners for sexual experiences. Unlike other forms of ENM where you might develop ongoing individual connections, swinging is primarily about couples meeting other couples for sexual play. You're doing this together, as a team.

The key distinction: this isn't about forming separate relationships outside your partnership. It's about enhancing your existing relationship through shared sexual experiences with other couples.

Swingers meet other couples and switch partners for sexual activities. This often happens in the same room. Part of the appeal is sharing the experience with your primary partner, not sneaking off to fuck someone else in private. Though separate rooms can happen depending on everyone's comfort level and the specific situation.

There's usually a social component too. Many swinger couples become friends, hang out outside of sexual contexts, travel together, or attend lifestyle events. It's not just about showing up, fucking, and leaving; though that definitely happens too.

The Levels: What Everyone's Comfortable With

Soft Swap: Making out, oral sex, touching, and heavy petting; but no penetrative sex with the other couple. This is often where new couples start to test the waters and see how they feel about sharing sexual experiences. This is also a good introduction to ENM in general.

Full Swap: Everything goes, including penetrative sex. P in V, anal, whatever everyone's comfortable with and excited about. No sexual activities are off-limits based on arbitrary swinging rules.

These aren't permanent categories. Couples might start soft and work up to full swap, or they might stick with soft swap indefinitely. Some couples might be full swap with certain people but only soft swap with others, depending on attraction and comfort levels.

For many couples, swinging enhances their primary relationship rather than threatening it. You're exploring sexuality together, meeting new people as a unit, and often the shared experiences create excitement that carries back into your relationship.

It can also scratch the itch for sexual variety without the emotional complexity of polyamory or the individual autonomy of open relationships. You're not managing multiple relationships or dating independently. You're having adventures together.

This lifestyle requires solid communication, clear boundaries, and genuine enthusiasm from both partners. One person dragging a reluctant partner into swinging is a recipe for disaster. Both people need to actively want this, not just be willing to tolerate it for their partner's sake.

Hotwifing: The Art of Coming Home

Not to be confused with cuckolding. Hotwifing gets lumped in with cuckolding, but they're different beasts entirely. While cuckolding often involves the husband being denigrated and humiliated.

Hotwifing is about shared excitement and reconnection. Also, despite the name, this dynamic works with any gender configuration. Husbands can absolutely be the ones going out and reporting back.

In hotwifing, one partner (traditionally the wife) has sexual encounters outside the relationship, then comes home to share the experience with their primary partner. The setup can vary wildly depending on the couple's comfort level and preferences.

Some couples go all out: elaborate dinners with all three people to check chemistry, vet the potential partner for safety, and make sure everyone's comfortable. Others keep it simple: "Hey honey, I'm going on a date. I'll tell you all about it when I get home."

The key element is what happens after. When the sex is done, the partner comes home and gives a detailed play-by-play. The listening partner gets off on hearing every detail of their partner's sexual adventure.

The appeal varies, but there are some common themes:

Pride and possession: "My partner is so desirable that other people are desperate to fuck them." It's another way of showing off what you have.

Power dynamics: Some partners enjoy orchestrating the encounters. Deciding who their partner fucks and how. It's a control kink where they get off on directing their partner's sexual experiences.

Vicarious thrill: Living out sexual fantasies through their partner's experiences, hearing about adventures they might not have themselves.

Compersion: Many couples experience genuine joy and satisfaction from their partner's pleasure with others. It's not just sexual arousal. It's emotional happiness from seeing their partner fulfilled.

Confidence and empowerment: For the partner going out, being desired by multiple people can be incredibly confidence-boosting and sexually empowering. It's validation that extends beyond their primary relationship.

The voyeuristic-reclamation spectrum: Some partners are more turned on by the voyeuristic thrill of imagining or hearing about the encounter, others get off primarily on the "reclaiming" sex afterward, and many enjoy both elements.

Here's what makes hotwifing work for many couples: the coming home is as important as the going out. The partner who stayed home is turned on hearing about their partner's sexual adventures, and the reconnection sex that follows is often intense as hell.

For the partner who went out, it's genuinely a "coming home." Returning to their primary connection after exploring elsewhere. For the partner who stayed, there's often a reclamation element in reestablishing their sexual connection after their partner's adventure.

Some practical realities:

Managing jealousy: Despite the turn-on factor, jealousy and insecurity absolutely come up. Successful couples develop strategies for handling these moments. Whether it's immediate reassurance, processing conversations, or adjusting boundaries or practices when needed.

Finding and vetting partners: While this can be just swiping on dating apps, couples still need to screen for people who understand the dynamic, respect boundaries, and prioritize safety. Some prefer ongoing relationships with trusted partners, others enjoy the variety of new encounters.

Communication protocols: What gets shared, when, and in how much detail varies by couple. Some want every graphic detail immediately, others prefer a general summary later. Figuring out these preferences takes trial and error.

The evolution factor: These relationships often start casual but can develop emotional connections over time. Couples need to navigate when a fuck buddy starts feeling like something more and decide if that works for their relationship structure.

Scheduling and logistics: Real life intrudes. Coordinating these encounters around work, kids, family obligations, and your own relationship time requires serious time management skills.

Gender dynamics: When roles are reversed (hothusband scenarios), the dynamics shift significantly. Safety considerations are different, social reactions vary, and the power dynamics can play out differently.

Like all ethical non-monogamy, this only works with enthusiastic consent from everyone involved. No one's getting pimped out or coerced. The partner going out has to genuinely enjoy these encounters, not just tolerate them for their partner's kink. When it works, both partners are getting something meaningful out of the dynamic.

Cuckolding: Humiliation as Arousal

Cuckolding and hotwifing look similar on the surface. One partner fucking someone else while the other watches or knows about it. But cuckolding has a crucial additional element: humiliation. The cuckold (usually male, though not exclusively) gets erotically stimulated by being denigrated during their partner's sexual encounter.

This isn't about sharing excitement or pride like in hotwifing. It's about getting off on being told you're inadequate, watching someone else pleasure your partner "better" than you can, and being made to feel small or powerless. It's a humiliation kink, and like all kinks between consenting adults, it deserves respect rather than judgment.

The "bull" (the person brought in to fuck the cuckold's partner) isn't just there for sex. They're there to dominate and humiliate the cuckold too. This can happen in various ways:

Watching from the corner: The cuckold sits in a chair, maybe jerking off, while being forced to watch their partner get fucked by someone else.

Verbal humiliation: The bull talks down to the cuckold, making comments like "Look how much better I fuck your wife" or pointing out the cuckold's supposed inadequacies.

Size humiliation: A major component often involves the bull having a larger penis and making that central to the humiliation. "Look how much bigger I am than your pathetic little dick."

Feminization: Many cuckolds get off on being made to feel "less masculine" during the encounter. Being called names, treated as submissive, or even made to wear feminine clothing.

Cleanup duty: After the bull cums inside the partner, the cuckold is made to "clean up" licking the bull's cum out of their partner's pussy. This isn't required but is often an element.

Sexual submission: Some cuckolds are bisexual and enjoy being dominated by the bull as well, adding another layer of submission to the dynamic.

There are endless variations depending on what specific humiliation elements turn everyone on.

At first glance, this might seem extreme or psychologically damaging. But plenty of people discover they genuinely enjoy this dynamic from both sides. The arousal comes from the power exchange, the taboo nature of the situation, and yes, the humiliation itself.

For some people, being "forced" to watch their partner with someone else while being told they're inadequate hits exactly the right psychological buttons to create intense sexual arousal.

There are complex emotions involved here. Many cuckolds experience genuine jealousy and emotional pain alongside the arousal. This psychological cocktail of conflicting feelings; hurt, arousal, jealousy, excitement creates an intensity that's hard to explain but compelling as fuck for those wired this way.

There can also be a racial element involved; particularly involving BBC (Big Black Cocks) with white couples. This adds layers of taboo that some find arousing; however, it can also play into harmful racial stereotypes. It's controversial and problematic, but it does happen and pretending it doesn't exist won't help anyone understand what's actually happening in this kink. If this is going to be an element of the scene it is important to recognize the historical abuses that black men and women have endured, even if they are equally excited to engage in the game.

Experienced bulls understand that this is elaborate sexual theater, not actual emotional abuse. These scenes are negotiated beforehand to establish limits, boundaries, and safe words. Everyone knows what they're signing up for, and no one's trying to cause genuine psychological damage. It's so important to find bulls that understand that the humiliation is consensual and contained within the sexual encounter. It's role-playing, not real relationship destruction.

The Practicalities

Finding the right bull: This isn't just about finding someone willing to fuck. Couples need someone who understands the psychological dynamics, respects boundaries, and can deliver the right kind of domination without crossing into actual abuse.

The bull's perspective: Good bulls take this responsibility seriously. They're not just there to get off - they're facilitating a complex psychological scene for a couple. Many develop ongoing relationships with couples rather than one-off encounters.

Aftercare matters: What happens after the scene is crucial. Couples need to reconnect and process what just happened. The intense emotions stirred up don't just disappear when everyone gets dressed.

Long-term relationship impact: This kink can strengthen some relationships by fulfilling deep psychological needs, but it can also create unexpected emotional complications. Jealousy and humiliation don't always stay contained in the bedroom.

Stag/Vixen: The Voyeuristic Pride Dynamic

Stag/vixen is a subgenre of hotwifing with its own distinct flavor. While traditional hotwifing often involves the partner going out alone and reporting back, stag/vixen dynamics center around the husband (stag) being present during his wife's (vixen) encounters with other men.

The key difference is this isn't about humiliation, degradation, or even necessarily about intense reconnection afterward. It's a more focused dynamic built around "my wife is so fucking hot, everything she does turns me on."

There are a couple of appeals here:

Pure voyeuristic pleasure: The stag gets off on watching his partner in action. There's something incredibly arousing about seeing your partner from this new angle. Watching her techniques, her responses, her pleasure with someone else. She is a real-life porn star.

Pride without humiliation: Unlike cuckolding, there's no element of being "less than" the other man. The stag feels proud that he has such a desirable partner that other men want to fuck her. It's showing off, not being shown up.

In-the-moment arousal: While hotwifing often builds toward the reconnection afterward, stag/vixen is more about the immediate thrill of what's happening right now.

The stag's level of engagement varies depending on the couple's preferences and boundaries.

Observer mode: The stag watches from a chair or the side of the bed, maybe masturbating while his vixen and the bull go at it.

Director role: Some stags enjoy giving gentle (or not so gentle) direction. Suggesting positions, telling the vixen what to do, or guiding the encounter.

Limited participation: The stag might join in for specific acts (oral, touching) while the bull handles the main event, or take turns with different activities.

Photography/recording: Many stag/vixen couples enjoy capturing the encounter for later enjoyment (with everyone's consent, obviously).

This dynamic often works well for women who enjoy being the center of attention and sexual focus. The vixen gets to feel desired by multiple men simultaneously; both her partner and the bull are focused on her pleasure. She can also explore her exhibitionist side in a safe, controlled environment with her partner present. As well as enjoy the power dynamic of being the object of desire that two men are competing to please.

Some practicalities to consider

Finding the right bulls: Not every guy is comfortable performing with an audience or being directed. You need partners who understand they're part of a couple's shared fantasy.

Setting boundaries: Clear communication about what the stag can and can't do during encounters, what the vixen is comfortable with, and what the bull's role should be.

Logistics: Unlike solo hotwifing dates, these encounters require coordinating schedules and finding appropriate spaces where everyone can be comfortable.

Safety protocols: With multiple people involved, extra attention to sexual health testing, consent discussions, and safety planning becomes crucial.

There is an emotional reality as well.

Managing performance pressure: Both the vixen and bull might feel pressure to "perform" for the watching stag, which can affect natural sexual flow.

There can be jealousy in real-time: Unlike hotwifing where jealousy might hit later during the storytelling, stags might experience unexpected jealousy while watching, requiring immediate communication.

The comparison trap: Even without the humiliation element, stags might find themselves comparing their own performance to the bull's, which can create unexpected insecurity.

Relationship impact: Some couples find that watching together enhances their connection, while others discover it creates complications they didn't anticipate.

Cheating in ENM: When Having Permission Makes Betrayal Worse
Redefining Cheating

When your partners are already fucking other people, what does cheating even mean? In ENM relationships, cheating isn't about sexual or romantic exclusivity. It's about deception and boundary violations.

Cheating in ENM boils down to anything involving deceiving your partner about what you're doing and/or with whom you're doing it. It's breaking the agreements you've made together, whether that's about safer sex practices, emotional boundaries, or communication protocols.

Cheating in ENM hits different. ENM relationships require robust honesty, authenticity, and communication to function. Because jealousy and trust are such huge components of any relationship, having those violated within an ENM structure can be absolutely catastrophic. It can be equally as damaging as in monogamous relationships and sometimes worse.

What makes it particularly brutal is that there's explicit space for difficult conversations in ENM relationships. There's purposeful room made to talk about unmet needs, desires to explore new kinks, or interest in different types of connections or people. When these spaces exist but aren't used the betrayal hits harder and the damage lasts longer.

What ENM Cheating Actually Looks Like

Breaking safer sex agreements: Having unprotected sex when you've agreed to use barriers, or not getting tested as promised.

Hiding relationships: Keeping a connection secret when you've agreed to transparency about partners.

Violating emotional boundaries: Lying about developing romantic feelings with someone when you've agreed to keep things purely sexual, or vice versa.

Time and priority violations: Consistently prioritizing other partners over agreed-upon time with your primary partner, or breaking dates/commitments repeatedly.

Communication violations: Not disclosing information you've agreed to share. Or sharing information about your partner that they've asked you to keep private.

Boundary escalation: Gradually pushing past established boundaries without explicit renegotiation.

The "don't ask, don't tell" trap: Using DADT agreements to hide behavior you know your partner wouldn't be okay with.

Some of the particular cruelties of ENM betrayal:

"I gave you permission and you still lied": The betrayed partner trusted enough to open the relationship, making deception feel like a deeper violation of that trust.

"You had options and chose deception": Unlike monogamy where some people cheat because they feel trapped, ENM provides legitimate outlets for desires; making deception feel more intentional.

"Why did we bother making specific agreements?": ENM couples often spend months negotiating detailed agreements, making violations feel like deliberate dismissal of that collaborative work.

Meta-betrayal: Sometimes the cheating partner has encouraged their partner to be vulnerable about their jealousy and insecurity, then violates boundaries anyway. This betrays both the relationship agreements and the emotional vulnerability.

ENM cheating gets complicated because:

Agreements evolve: What you agreed to six months ago might not fit your current situation, but changing agreements requires communication, not unilateral deception.

Gray areas exist: Sometimes it's genuinely unclear whether something violates your agreements. These situations require immediate communication, not assumption.

Different relationship styles, different rules: What counts as cheating in hierarchical polyamory might be different from relationship anarchy agreements. Again, robust communication is key.

Emotional vs. logistical boundaries: Violating someone's emotional boundaries can be cheating even if you technically followed the "rules." For example: A couple agrees that they can have casual sexual encounters but should avoid "romantic" activities like staying overnight, meeting each other's families, or saying "I love you." The husband starts having regular sex with a coworker. He follows all the "rules;" no sleepovers, no family introductions, no love declarations. Instead, he starts texting her constantly throughout the day, sharing intimate details about his marriage problems, turning to her for emotional support instead of his wife, and prioritizing her needs when she's having a crisis. Technically, he hasn't broken any explicit agreements. But he's developed an emotional intimacy that his wife feels threatened by and that violates the spirit of their "casual only" boundary. His wife feels like he's having an emotional affair even though he never said "I love you" or spent the night. The wife's emotional boundary was about not being replaced as his primary emotional partner. Even though the logistical rules were followed, the emotional boundary got completely trampled. He created a deeper connection than what they agreed to, just without the obvious markers they'd tried to rule out.

This is why many ENM couples learn that you can't just make a list of prohibited activities. You have to understand and respect the emotional intentions behind the boundaries too. It's the spirit of the rule that matters.

Recovery & Repair: Possible, but Requires Some Heavy Lifting

Immediate transparency: Complete honesty about what happened, why, and with whom.

Taking responsibility: Acknowledging the violation without minimizing or blaming your partner's "rules" or jealousy. Own your shit.

Understanding the impact: Recognizing that you didn't just break an agreement. You violated the trust that makes ENM possible.

Rebuilding slowly: Trust reconstruction often means returning to more restrictive agreements while you prove reliability again.

Professional help: Many couples need therapy specifically focused on betrayal trauma and rebuilding trust in non-monogamous contexts.

Having permission to be with other people doesn't eliminate the possibility of betrayal. It just changes what betrayal looks like. The foundation of ENM is trust and communication. When that foundation gets damaged through deception, the repair work is just as complex and painful as in any other relationship structure.

The difference is that in ENM, you had alternatives to betrayal. That makes the choice to deceive even harder to understand and forgive.

Compersion: The Holy Grail That You Don't Actually Need

Compersion is feeling genuine joy and happiness when your partner is experiencing romantic or sexual pleasure with someone else. Not just being okay with it, not just tolerating it, but actually feeling positive emotions about your partner's connections with others.

It's often called the "opposite of jealousy," though that's not entirely accurate. Jealousy and compersion can actually coexist. You might feel both happy for your partner and insecure about yourself in the same moment. Feelings are funny, huh?

In many ENM communities, compersion gets treated like the ultimate goal. The enlightened state that proves you're "doing polyamory right." This creates enormous pressure and shame for people who don't naturally feel joy about their partner fucking other people.

Let's be clear: **you do not need to feel compersion to have successful ENM relationships.** It's not a requirement, it's not a measure of your growth, and it's not something you should fake.

When people do experience compersion, it might show up as: genuine excitement when your partner talks about a great date or amazing sex with someone else. Or feeling proud that your partner is desired and appreciated by others. Joy in seeing your partner happy even when that happiness comes from another relationship. It could be sexual arousal from hearing about your partner's encounters (though this overlaps with other kinks). Or the warm fuzzy feelings about your partner's other relationships enriching their life

In reality though, it's complicated.

It's not consistent: You might feel compersion with one metamour but not another. Or feel it sometimes but not always.

It's not immediate: Some people develop compersion over time as they build security and trust. Others never do, and that's fine.

It's not universal: Even people who experience compersion don't feel it about every aspect of their partner's other relationships.

It can be situational: You might feel compersion when you're in a good mood, but jealousy when you're having a rough day.

Many people in successful ENM relationships never experience true compersion. Instead, they might feel:

Neutral acceptance: "My partner is on a date. Cool, I'm going to watch Netflix."

Mild positive feelings: Not joy, exactly, but general good vibes about your partner's happiness.

Intellectual appreciation: Understanding that your partner's other relationships are good for them, even if you don't feel emotionally excited about it.

Focus on your own stuff: Being genuinely busy with and excited about your own life while your partner does theirs.

All of these are completely valid ways to practice ENM.

Pretending to feel compersion when you don't is a recipe for disaster. Your partner will likely sense the disconnect, and you'll build resentment about having to perform emotions you don't feel. It's much better to honestly say "I'm working on being okay with this" or "I don't feel joy about it, but I support your happiness" than to fake enthusiasm you don't have.

Cultivating Compersion (Without Forcing It)

If you're interested in developing compersion, some things that might help:

- Focus on your partner's happiness rather than the specific sexual or romantic details
- Build security in your own relationship so other connections feel less threatening. This might mean being more intentional about going on dates or making time for each other.
- Develop your own fulfilling connections or interests so you're not sitting around stewing while your partner has fun
- Practice gratitude for what your partner's other relationships give them that you might not be able or interested in providing
- Remember the benefits that your partner's happiness and fulfillment bring to your relationship

Compersion is a nice bonus, not a necessity. What matters is that you feel loved, valued, and secure in your relationship(s). Whether you get there through compersion, neutral acceptance, or just really good communication and boundaries is entirely up to you.

Don't let anyone tell you that you're not "evolved" enough if you don't feel joy about your partner's other relationships. ENM success is measured by whether everyone involved feels happy and fulfilled, not by whether you've achieved some specific emotional state.

Dealing with Jealousy: The Universal Challenge

The fucking reality is jealousy is the bane of all relationships, monogamous or non-monogamous. Whole books are written about this subject (see appendix for detailed resources), but here's what you need to understand: jealousy will happen. Even in the most secure relationships, even with the most communication, even when everyone's doing everything "right." Feeling jealous doesn't mean your relationship is flawed. It's a normal human emotion. It's okay.

At its heart, jealousy is insecurity wrapped in fear. A person feels jealous because they're scared of being replaced, not being good enough, losing their relationship, or discovering their partner likes someone else more. It's fundamentally the fear that "my partner isn't satisfied with me, which means something is wrong with me."

When so much of our identity gets wrapped up in being in a committed relationship, these fears become absolutely terrifying. The threat feels existential. It's not just losing a partner, but losing who we are.

Under traditional relationship models, the solution to jealousy is simple: the other partner changes. Changes their desires, their fantasies, their actions. Changes who they talk to, where they go, how often they check in. Restrict, limit, control.

This solution is fundamentally broken and unsustainable in both monogamous and non-monogamous relationships. It doesn't address the root cause. The jealous partner never actually works on their own fears and insecurities. It's like bailing water out of a boat instead of fixing the hole. It's also unfair to put the responsibility for one's emotions on another person. One person's insecurity becomes someone else's problem to manage. Also, it just doesn't work. No matter how much you compromise to alleviate your partner's jealousy, it will never be enough. The insecurity will just find new things to focus on. Which will create resentment. The partner doing the restricting will eventually feel controlled and resentful.

What Actually Helps

Collaboration, not control: Work together to understand the jealousy rather than eliminate its triggers. Learn to ride the waves of the emotion rather than run from them. Don't fight the tide, surf it. I've said before feelings lie to us. Jealousy feels like an existential threat but it's really not. Once you look it in the eye, it's just like every other feeling.

Reassurance with honesty: Listen to your partner's fears and provide genuine reassurance where you can. Never lie to a jealous person, that will make it worse, but you can share good truths. How you see them, how much you love them, what makes them special to you.

Emotional responsibility: The jealous partner needs to own their feelings while the other partner offers support. Blaming your partner for your insecurity is not only misplaced, but also just mean, man.

Vulnerability and communication: Sharing fears requires vulnerability. Creating safe spaces for these conversations is crucial for both partners. It's very easy to become defensive when a jealous partner is telling you about their feelings because we are programed to interpret that as them saying you're doing something wrong. It takes practice and time to unlearn these assumptions on both sides.

Practical Jealousy Management

Identify triggers: What specific scenarios, times, or situations tend to bring up jealousy? Understanding patterns helps you prepare.

Develop self-soothing skills: The jealous partner needs tools for managing their anxiety when it hits. Breathing exercises, grounding techniques, self-talk strategies.

Create check-in protocols: Regular relationship maintenance conversations, not crisis management when jealousy explodes.

Invest in your primary relationship: One of the things that fuels jealousy is when a couple stops going on dates with each other and most of the dressing up and going out is with other people. Make time to invest in each other and your time together. If you're dating other people, don't forget to date your partner too.

Set realistic timelines: Jealousy doesn't disappear overnight. It's often a long process of building security and trust. It will continue to occur even after you think you've "fixed it." New relationships start the process all over again. Even for monogamous people.

Know when to get help: Sometimes working through jealousy requires professional support. Don't be afraid of couples therapy, in fact go before you "need to." It is important to find a therapist that is versed in ENM concepts. Unfortunately, many therapists also subscribe to the standard narrative that doesn't really work for ENM relationships.

Here's the thing, jealousy can actually be useful information. It often points to real needs that aren't being met. The need for more quality time, better communication, increased intimacy, or addressing relationship issues that have nothing to do with other partners.

Working through jealousy together, when done with care and commitment, can really strengthen relationships. But it requires both partners to show up authentically and do the hard emotional work.

When Jealousy Becomes Destructive

Controlling behavior: Demanding to read texts, forbidding certain activities, or isolating partners from friends.

Emotional manipulation: Using tears, anger, or threats to control your partner's behavior.

Stalking or surveillance: Checking up on partners without their consent or following them, online or in person.

Verbal or physical aggression: Jealousy that escalates to abuse is never acceptable.

If jealousy manifests in these ways, it's time to step back from ENM and get professional help. ENM amplifies existing relationship dynamics. So if control and manipulation are already present, adding more partners will make things worse, not better.

CHAPTER NINE

Problems

Sexual Problems: It's Not All Fun & Games

In sex, as in life, problems arise. Just like we wouldn't expect there to be no challenges in life, we shouldn't expect there to be no challenges in bed. Here are a few of the most common challenges people run into during sex.

Getting In Your Head

The number one buzzkill is getting self-conscious. You start worrying about how you look, sound, smell, or perform. You're wondering if your partner is enjoying it or secretly judging you. This mental spiral can absolutely fuck up what should be a good time.

Often this stems from our society's tendency to body shame. Mass media has spent decades telling us our bodies are wrong. Too fat, too thin, too hairy, not hairy enough, boobs too small, ass not big enough, dick too small, whatever. This shit follows us into the bedroom and kills the mood.

Reality Check: Your partner chose to be naked with you. They're not conducting a detailed inspection looking for flaws. They're trying to have a good time with someone they're attracted to. Hi, that's you!

Practical approaches include keeping the lighting dim but on since darkness might feel safer, but it also disconnects you from the experience and we like to see how much our partner is enjoying us. Focus on what feels good, not how you think you look. Remember that confidence is sexy as hell. Own your body and your pleasure. Whatever your body type there are people who are into it, they may not get a lot of airtime in mainstream media, but they do exist! If negative thoughts creep in, redirect to physical sensations. What you're feeling, touching, experiencing. Consider that your partner probably has their own insecurities and isn't scrutinizing you nearly as much as you think.

For Penis Owners

The biggest anxieties usually centers around two things: "Am I getting hard enough fast enough?" or "Am I big enough?"

Let's take hardness first. Sure, there are meds for erections, but they work best when the problem is physical (like age-related performance decline). When it's psychological, the pathways to arousal are different and don't entirely rely on the enzymes those meds target.

Specifically, PDE-5 (phosphodiesterase type 5) is an enzyme your body secretes after you cum to tell your penis it doesn't need to be hard anymore. Meds like Viagra are PDE-5 inhibitors. They reduce the amount of PDE-5 telling your penis to back down. As you age your body secretes PDE-5 earlier than necessary. Meds like Viagra inhibit this process, reducing the amount of PDE-5 in your blood stream. If the reason you can't get hard is because you're in your head and thinking about it too much, Viagra won't help. Being in your head causes a stress response that inhibits your erection, not PDE-5. However, if you're getting older and you're nervous about it, taking some Viagra can give you some peace of mind that physically it's not an issue. Some people call it swinger insurance.

As for size anxiety: the average erect penis is actually between 5 and 6 inches. Because porn only employs actors with above-average sizes, we think that's the standard, but it's not! Porn dicks are like porn everything else, selected for visual impact, not reality.

Here's the thing: if your partner wants something bigger to fill them up, toys are your friend. Don't let your ego get in the way of good sex. A smaller penis plus a well-chosen toy can be way more fun than a big dick with no game. Honestly, if you're on the smaller side, you're probably perfectly sized for anal play. No warm-up required!

The reality is that most vaginas are only sensitive in the first few inches anyway, and technique matters way more than size. A smaller penis that knows what it's doing will often beat a big one that just jackhammers away. Focus on what you can control. Your skills, your enthusiasm, and your willingness to use whatever tools make the experience better for everyone involved.

For Vagina Owners

Similar anxiety happens around getting wet. Good news: lube is your best friend for sexy times, and it doesn't matter what mechanism is holding you back. Don't be shy about it. For vagina owners the problem is more often a worry about reaching orgasm.

Common Sexual Problems and Solutions

Cumming Too Slow

More common for vagina owners, but again, can affect anyone. Worrying about it makes you less aroused and makes it even harder to reach orgasm.   Stay Present. Focus on what feels good in the moment. Don't be shy about giving directions to guide your partner. Remember that going into sexual activities with a goal-oriented mindset is a great way to ruin the fun. Make the goal the pleasurable journey, not the destination. Sometimes you'll cum, sometimes you won't, and that's okay. Fun, pleasurable sex that doesn't end in orgasm is still successful sex.

Cumming Too Fast

Usually affects penis owners but can happen to anyone. The more you worry about it, the worse it gets. The average time it takes for men to cum is about 3-7 minutes, but this number is incredibly influenced by outside factors like age, familiarity with partner, arousal level, recent orgasms, and more. My point is the idea that a fuck session has to last an hour is unrealistic. That's fantasy porn land.

If you're worried about cumming too soon or before your partner, focus on getting them off first with oral sex, toys, or fingers, then use your dick after they've already cum. Or use your dick for a bit, then if you're about to cum, stop and switch things up. Move to oral or change positions to give yourself time to cool down.

Same goes if you happen to cum earlier than you'd like. There are still plenty of other things you can do that don't involve your dick to make your partner feel good. Use your hands and mouth and don't be shy about it. Confidence is sexy. Whatever you do, don't fall asleep after orgasm if your partner hasn't cum yet. Rally, my friend! Use what you've got and provide that pleasure. Again, not with a goal-oriented mindset but a "I want to make you feel good like you made me feel good" kind of mindset. If they don't end up cumming, don't take it personally, they may have been in their head.

One of the methods to address these things are pelvic floor exercises. Kegel exercises strengthen the muscle you use to control your pee. For penis owners, this is the same muscle that helps control ejaculation (which is separate from orgasm, though they usually happen together). For vagina owners, Kegels strengthen vaginal walls, increasing sensation during penetration. Fun fact: you can do these anywhere. In a boring business meeting? Knock out some reps while fantasizing about later.

Medication Side Effects

A lot of common medications can fuck with your sex life, and doctors don't always warn you about this shit.

Common culprits include antidepressants (especially SSRIs) which can kill libido and make orgasm difficult or impossible. Incidentally, this can be helpful if your problem is cumming too fast. Birth control with hormonal versions can tank sex drive, which is kinda ironic that the drug you take in order to have anxiety free sex takes away your desire to have sex… life is funny sometimes. There are lots of different types of birth control, find one that works for you. Blood pressure meds can affect erections and can be dangerous in combination with PDE-5 inhibitors. Antihistamines can dry you out everywhere, including down there and make you too tired to want to play.

What you can do for these is talk to your doctor about alternative meds, adjustments, or timing. Sometimes switching medications or adjusting doses helps. Just don't suffer in silence or stop taking necessary meds without medical guidance.

Hormonal Changes

Your hormones are like the backstage crew of your sex life; when they're off, everything feels off.

Common hormone-related issues include menopause where estrogen drops, which can cause vaginal dryness, reduced libido, and painful sex. Pregnancy and postpartum periods mean hormones are all over the place, plus you're exhausted and your body has changed. Testosterone decline happens with age for everyone, affecting libido and energy. Your menstrual cycle naturally causes libido to fluctuate throughout the month. Stress means cortisol can suppress the happy sex hormones. The point is there are factors at play beyond what's happening in the moment.

Hormone replacement therapy might help. Talk to a doctor, not TikTok. Good lube is essential. Be patient with your body during life transitions. Consider that this is normal biological stuff, not a personal failing.

Anatomy 101: Know Your Equipment

Shocking how many people don't know basic anatomy. Here's what you need to know:

For Vagina Owners

The clitoris has about 8,000 nerve endings (twice as many as a penis) and extends internally. What you see is just the tip. The visible part is usually nestled under a protective hood and depending on normal variations of bodies it can be helpful to use your hands to spread the labia and expose it more fully. Be careful though, it has a lot of nerve endings, too much stimulation can be more painful than fun. Additionally, the clitoris extends down the sides of the vagina as well, looking a bit like an upside down wishbone. These clitoral sides can also be stimulated by rubbing or licking the sides of the vagina.

The proverbial G-spot is about 1-2 inches inside the vaginal opening, on the front (top) wall. It feels like a slightly ridged bump. It's actually part of the clitoris, just behind a lot more padding. People often say the orgasm from the visible clitoris and from the buried G-spot feel different. Different people prefer one or the other, but both are normal.

Vaginal lubrication comes from blood flow to the area, not from a specific gland, just like with penises. And squirting (female ejaculation) does not mean an orgasm has occurred, though it can accompany one and not everyone squirts when the cum. This is another myth given to us by porn. Also, the vagina is self-cleaning. Don't douche or use harsh soaps inside, it's not necessary and causes irritation.

For Penis Owners

Erections happen when blood flows into spongy tissue and gets trapped there. How that blood flows and stays trapped involves getting out of your body's way and/or adjusting the way your body uses enzymes and hormones.

The frenulum (underside of the head) is often the most sensitive part. This is actually the male equivalent of the clit. The head is the clit and the foreskin is the hood. Before the second trimester of pregnancy, all fetuses are female and have the coding for female genitalia; if there is a Y chromosome it fires in the 2nd trimester and the cells that would become a vagina, clitoris, and ovaries become a shaft, head (with foreskin), and testes.

Circumcised vs. uncircumcised affects sensitivity and may require different techniques. Uncircumcised penises have the foreskin, which is like the protective hood for the clitoris. Sometimes you might have to manually move it aside to get to the good stuff.

Ejaculation and orgasm are separate events that usually happen together but don't have to. For example, the prostate is often called the male G-spot because you can rub it like the female G-spot and get an intense orgasm but not necessarily ejaculate. It's located about 1-2 inches inside the rectum. Which is another reason straight guys need to get over the fear of being perceived gay if they indulge in butt stuff. It's doesn't matter who is doing the stimulating, it feels fucking amazing when done right.

For Everyone

Arousal takes time, rushing kills the mood. Foreplay, flirting, making out are all great ways to increase that arousal. The anticipation makes the actual event so much better. This can also really help with getting out of your head. If you find yourself struggling with your mind, moving back into making out, flirting, or exploring sensations can take the performance pressure off a bit and ground you in physical sensation allowing that arousal to happen naturally again. Foreplay isn't just foreplay, it's also anxiety management; and grounding yourself isn't just mindfulness bullshit, these are practical ways to get your mind and body back on track.

Different people have different sensitive spots. Explore and communicate. Anatomy varies widely. What works for one person might not work for another so have fun exploring and communicating what you like and discovering new sensations.

When Sex Hurts

Pain during sex, like life, usually means stop. Unless it's a kink you're exploring consensually.

Bodies come in all sizes, and trying to fit large items into small spaces can cause pain. Depending on severity, warming up can help (essential for anal play). Sometimes no amount of warm-up will make something fit. If you have a particularly tight or small space, consider talking to a medical professional about training or stretching options.

Pain during anal means stop immediately. The tissues around your anus are sensitive (which is why anal can be amazing regardless of orientation) but also thin. Tears happen, and they're a major risk factor for STI transmission because those tiny tears create entry points for infections. Also tears hurt! Butts need to be warmed up and lubed up. Reapply lube before you think you need to. The vagina creates its own lube; butts do not and rely on you to add it in there. This is never shown in porn but believe me it's happening in between cuts and behind the scenes. If you're using toys with butt play, they **MUST** have a flared base otherwise you will end up in the emergency room and they will talk about you in the break room.

Reclaiming Sexuality After Trauma

This is very important work that can be incredibly cathartic and empowering. Sexual trauma can fuck with your relationship to your body, pleasure, and intimacy in ways that feel overwhelming, but healing is absolutely possible.

Find a sex-positive therapist who specializes in trauma work. This will be an ongoing journey with its own ups and downs, and you deserve professional support through it. Look specifically for therapists trained in trauma-informed approaches, not just general counselors who might not understand the complexities of sexual healing.

Some things to expect: Progress isn't linear. You might feel great one day and triggered the next. That's normal, not failure. Your body might react in ways that surprise you, like sudden panic during what should be pleasurable moments. These reactions are your nervous system defaulting to protecting you, not something you're doing wrong.

Practical approaches that can help: Start slow and prioritize consent. Including consent with yourself. You get to change your mind, stop, or say no at any point. Practice body awareness through non-sexual touch first. Masturbation can be a way to reconnect with your body on your terms. Communicate with partners about what you need, including specific words or actions that might be triggering.

Remember: There's no timeline for "getting over it" and no finish line where you're suddenly "normal" again. Healing looks different for everyone. The goal isn't to forget what happened or to have the same relationship with sex you had before. It's to create a new relationship with your body and sexuality that feels safe and authentic to who you are now.

Stay present, communicate openly, and remember that good sex is about connection and pleasure, not performance metrics. Your head can be your biggest enemy or your greatest ally. You're not broken, and your trauma doesn't define your sexual future.

CHAPTER TEN

STIs

There are many hundreds of other Sexually Transmitted Infections (STIs) a person can acquire but these are the most common. Since this is a simple sex ed book, I'm going to direct you to other sources for more detailed explanations of all the other boogers you can contract.

HIV/AIDS: From Boogieman to Manageable

HIV/AIDS used to be everyone's biggest sexual health nightmare, and honestly, that fear still lingers even though science has completely changed the game. The reality is that people living with HIV can have full, complete lives thanks to incredible advances in treatment. Modern antiretroviral medications are so effective that people who maintain undetectable viral loads literally cannot transmit HIV sexually. That's the "undetectable = un-transmittable" or U=U principle, and it's fucking revolutionary.

But let's talk prevention, because that's where things get really interesting. PrEP (Pre-Exposure Prophylaxis) is a daily pill that dramatically reduces your risk of HIV infection. According to the CDC, when taken consistently, PrEP reduces your risk of getting HIV from sex by about 99%. That's comparable to condom effectiveness for HIV specifically.

Here's the catch though, and this is important; PrEP only protects against HIV. It won't do shit for chlamydia, gonorrhea, syphilis, herpes, or any of the other infections you can pick up during unprotected sex. That's why I still recommend using condoms. PrEP gives you killer HIV protection, but you need that barrier method for everything else.

Syphilis: The Persistent Bastard

Syphilis feels like one of those diseases we should have eradicated by now with vaccines, right? Well, here's the frustrating truth: while treatment is incredibly effective, we still don't have a vaccine for it. And unfortunately, it's not as rare as we'd like. Syphilis rates have actually been climbing in recent years, which is some bullshit we need to take seriously.

The good news is that syphilis is totally treatable, especially when caught early. The tricky part is recognizing the symptoms because they can be sneaky as hell. The first stage usually shows up as painless sores (called chancres) on your genitals, anus, or mouth. Not your palms. These sores are highly contagious and can appear anywhere the bacteria entered your body.

If left untreated, syphilis progresses through stages. The second stage can cause rashes (including on your palms and soles of your feet), flu-like symptoms, and other nasty stuff. Here's where it gets serious. If you let this fucker progress to late-stage syphilis, it can cause irreversible damage to your brain, heart, and other organs. We're talking dementia, psychosis, and other life-altering complications.

The bottom line? Don't fuck around with syphilis. If you notice any suspicious sores or symptoms, get tested. Early treatment with antibiotics (usually penicillin) will knock it out completely.

Gonorrhea and Chlamydia: The Common Culprits

Gonorrhea and chlamydia are the most common bacterial STIs out there. They're like the uninvited guests that show up to way too many sexual encounters. The good news? Antibiotics are incredibly effective at treating both of these infections when caught early.

Here's the tricky part that trips people up. These infections are sneaky as hell. They often don't cause any symptoms at all, especially in people with vaginas. You could be walking around feeling perfectly fine while unknowingly passing the infection to partners or letting it quietly damage your reproductive system.

When symptoms do show up, they might include painful urination, unusual discharge, or pelvic pain. But don't wait for symptoms, that's a losing game. If you're sexually active with multiple partners, regular testing is absolutely essential. We're talking every 3-6 months, or whenever you have unprotected sex with a new partner.

Left untreated, both gonorrhea and chlamydia can cause serious complications like pelvic inflammatory disease (PID), which can lead to infertility or chronic pain. In rare cases, they can even cause life-threatening infections that spread throughout your body.

The bottom line: these are totally preventable and treatable, but only if you're proactive about testing. Don't assume you're in the clear just because you feel fine.

Herpes: The Hard Truth

Here's the thing about herpes that's gonna blow your mind. In the U.S., most people already have HSV-1, the oral version of herpes. We're talking about 53% of adults age 19-49, depending on age group. These infections typically cause cold sores on the lips and inside the mouth, but here's the kicker, most people who carry the virus don't have any symptoms at all. They're walking around completely unaware they have it.

So, the idea that you can avoid herpes? That's kinda ridiculous because you probably already have it. If you don't have HSV-1, there's a decent chance you might pick it up. HSV-2 (the genital version) occurs in about 1 in 8.

Now here's where it gets interesting: HSV-1 and HSV-2 aren't stuck to their "preferred" locations. HSV-1 can absolutely cause genital herpes through oral sex, and HSV-2 can cause oral herpes, though that's less common. In fact, HSV-1 is becoming a major cause of genital herpes, especially among younger people. The virus doesn't give a shit about what we call it. It just wants to find a nice mucous membrane to call home.

The good news is that if you already have HSV-1 orally, you're pretty well protected against getting HSV-1 genitally. Your body's immune response recognizes the virus and says "nah, we're good." However, you can still get HSV-2 genitally even if you have HSV-1 orally.

For folks who do get outbreaks, whether it's cold sores or genital herpes, there are antiviral medications that work really well. You can take them daily to prevent outbreaks altogether, or situationally when you feel an outbreak coming on. The meds help it end sooner and be way less painful. Herpes has been stigmatized way out of proportion to its actual health impact. For most people, it's an occasional inconvenience, not a life-altering condition. The emotional impact of the diagnosis is often worse than the physical symptoms.

Usually, the first outbreak is the worst, and for most it's once or twice a year that outbreaks occur. For those with more frequent outbreaks there are daily antiviral meds you can take. Of course, talk to your health care provider, I'm not a doctor.

As for transmission, technicality the virus can "shed" meaning be transmitted at anytime. However, it is rare for the virus to be transmitted when there is no visible outbreak. So, if you're worried about it, all you need to do is look at your potential partner and see if there are any sores. Pretty simple. Now, it's pretty hot to tease or build the anticipation by getting your face really close to your partner, those little electric tingles that happen when the distance closes. Take the time to appreciate their scent and compliment their appearance. This also gives you some time to notice if there are any questionable bumps or sores.

The important takeaway here is that people with herpes can absolutely have normal, healthy sex lives. Antiviral medications, condoms, and communication with partners make transmission risk manageable.

The Bottom Line: Don't Let Fear Kill Your Fun

While STIs exist and should absolutely be on your radar, don't let the fear factor stop you from enjoying your sex life. We've got solid tools to significantly reduce your risk: condoms, dental dams, PrEP for HIV prevention, and even DoxyPEP (doxycycline post-exposure prophylaxis) which can help prevent bacterial STIs like chlamydia, gonorrhea, and syphilis when taken after potential exposure.

But here's something just as important as safer sex practices: paying attention to who you're fucking. Does this person practice safer sex with other partners? Do they care as much about not spreading infections as they do about not getting them? Are they getting tested regularly? Do they communicate openly about their sexual health?

These aren't just medical questions. They're character questions. Someone who's cavalier about your health probably isn't someone you want to be intimate with anyway.

Remember, you get to decide who and what activities you engage with, and you can draw the line anywhere you want. Maybe you're comfortable with certain risks with a long-term partner but not with someone new. Maybe you require recent test results before any sexual contact. Maybe you're okay with oral sex but want barriers for penetrative sex. Whatever your boundaries are, they're valid.

The goal isn't to eliminate all risk. That's impossible unless you're celibate. The goal is to make informed decisions that let you enjoy sex while protecting your health and peace of mind.

CHAPTER ELEVEN

For Further Exploration

Resources: Build Your Own Sexual Library

Thanks for sticking through all that info! Hopefully it was both informative and enjoyable. Sex and sexuality is a subject that just gets more and more interesting the deeper you dive in. These are some of my favorite sources of information. By no means is this an exhaustive list, but it's a solid place to start.

Go forth and build your own sexual library, your future self (and your partners) will thank you for it.

Ethical Non-Monogamy:

- The Ethical Slut by Janet Hardy & Dossie Easton
- Opening Up by Tristan Taormino
- Mating in Captivity by Esther Perel
- Sex at Dawn by Christopher Ryan and Cacilda Jethá.
- The Anxious Person's Guide to Non-Monogamy by Lola Phoenix
- Relationship Anarchy, by Juan Carlos & Perez Cortez
- More Than Two: A Practical Guide to Ethical Polyamory By Franklin Veaus, Janet Hardy, Tatiana Gill
- Polysecure by Jessica Fern
- The Polyamory Toolkit by Dan Williams and Dawn Williams

Kink:

- The Topping Book by Janet Hardy & Dossie Easton
- The Bottoming Book by Janet Hardy & Dossie Easton
- The Ultimate Guide to Prostrate Pleasure by Charlie Glickman
- The Dominance Playbook by Anton Pulmen
- Caring About Aftercare: Thesis Presentation of Initial Findings, by Sage Fuentes

LGBTQ

- Sex Matters for Women
- Becoming a Visible Man
- Queer America: A People's GLBT History of the United States by Vicki L. Eaklor
- American Savage, by Dan Savage
- If I Was Your Girl, by Meredith Russo

Positions, Technique & General Info:

- The Kama Sutra
- Good Sex, by Jessica Graham
- Sexual Intelligence, by Marty Klein, Phd
- She Comes First, by Ian Kerner
- The Joy of Sex by Alex Comfort, Phd
- The Art of Going Down, by Elizabeth Cramer
- The G-Spot series, by Percy Ella

Porn:

- Best Women's Erotica: various volumes by various authors
- My Secret Garden by Nancy Friday
- Make Love Not Porn, TED Talks, Cindy Gallop
- Xconfessions.com
- Erika Lust

Podcasts:

- Sex Nerd Sandra
- Sex With Emily
- Open Late
- Manwhore
- Sex Out Loud w/ Tristan Taormino
- We Gotta Thing